P9-CJV-203

Neurasthenic Nation

Critical Issues in Health and Medicine

Edited by Rima D. Apple, University of Wisconsin–Madison,
and Janet Golden, Rutgers University, Camden

Growing criticism of the U.S. health care system is coming from consumers, politicians, the media, activists, and health care professionals. Critical Issues in Health and Medicine is a collection of books that explores these contemporary dilemmas from a variety of perspectives, among them political, legal, historical, sociological, and comparative, and with attention to crucial dimensions such as race, gender, ethnicity, sexuality, and culture.

For a list of titles in the series, see the last page of the book.

Neurasthenic Nation

America's Search for Health, Happiness, and Comfort, 1869–1920

David G. Schuster

Rutgers University Press

New Brunswick, New Jersey, and London

Library of Congress Cataloging-in-Publication Data

Schuster, David G., 1969–
    Neurasthenic nation : America's search for health, happiness, and comfort, 1869–1920 /
David G. Schuster.
        p. ; cm. — (Critical issues in health and medicine)
    Includes bibliographical references and index.
    ISBN 978-0-8135-5131-9 (hardcover : alk. paper)
    1. Neurasthenia—United States—History—19th century.   2. Neurasthenia—United
States—History—20th century.   3. Americans—Health and hygiene—History—19th century.
4. Americans—Health and hygiene—History—20th century.   5. Industrial revolution—
Health aspects—United States.   I. Title.   II. Series: Critical issues in health and medicine.
    [DNLM: 1. Neurasthenia—history—United States.   2. History, 19th Century—United
States.   3. History, 20th Century—United States. WM 11 AA1]
    RC552.N5S38   2011
    362.196′852800973—dc22

                                                                          2010049937

A British Cataloging-in-Publication record for this book is available from the British Library.

Visit our Web site: http://rutgerspress.rutgers.edu

Manufactured in the United States of America

For my parents, John and Eleanor Schuster

Contents

Illustrations

Preface and Acknowledgments

This project began as an attempt to understand how Americans developed a sense of what it means to be a "normal" person. The question of what constitutes "normal" has intrigued me for most of my adult life. As an undergraduate I spent a year studying abroad in Scotland, a wonderful experience but one in which I occasionally felt out of sorts and alienated from those around me. Similar feelings came back years later when I moved from my home in California to teach at a school outside of Istanbul. I realized that I was not normal by local standards—I was an *yabancı*, a foreigner—and I was surprised how distressed this sometimes made me feel.

But what really got me thinking about what it meant to be normal was when three close friends were diagnosed with chronic health disorders as adults, two with bipolar disorder and one with fibromyalgia. These were people who had helped shaped my understanding of what it meant to be normal—I had known them since junior high school—and to learn that they were suffering from abnormal conditions was disorienting and made me doubt what I had previously taken for granted. However, their diagnoses had the opposite effect on them. Each related to me how her diagnosis helped bring order to her life by explaining what were otherwise confusing mood swings and chronic pain, experiences that had made at least one question her own sanity. For two of these friends, such diagnoses made it possible to look back and make sense of events and relationships that had troubled them for years.

In graduate school, I made it my goal to trace how Americans have come to develop a sense of what it is to be a normal person. As with most projects, this one hinged on finding a manageable way of approach. I had the privilege of having Mary O. Furner as my graduate advisor, and during one of our initial meetings, in which she patiently listened to me ramble on about culture, health, and the meaning of being normal, she interrupted to ask "Where does neurasthenia fit into it all?" My response was "What is neurasthenia?"

As it turns out, neurasthenia was the topic that made it manageable to bring together American history, culture, health, and what it means for people to think of themselves as normal. America's experience with neurasthenia encouraged people to look to happiness and comfort as the bellwethers of being of normal health. People who feel happy and comfortable probably think their health is pretty good. However, persons suffering from depression and pain will probably consider themselves sick, despite having normal temperature, pulse, and lab results.

Many persons have helped me on this project. I first must thank the woman who led me to the topic and stayed with me for the duration: Mary O. Furner. Professor Furner challenged me when I became complacent, showed compassion when I needed it, modeled what it meant to be a fine teacher as well as an erudite scholar, and endured my sometimes fanciful understanding of things. Thank you.

My history colleagues at Indiana University–Purdue University Fort Wayne (IPFW) have proven themselves wonderful friends as well as willing critics, and this book benefited greatly from their support and feedback. Barbara Blauvelt, Christine K. Erickson, Bernd Fischer, James A. Haw, Suzanne M. LaVere, Ann Livschiz, Richard Weiner—thank you all very much.

This project also owes a great deal to those who have taken an interest in it over the years, have provided invaluable commentary, and have helped me clarify my thoughts. Special thanks to Michael Osborne, Eric W. Boyle, Heidi Brevik, Sandra Dawson, Anita Guerrini, Rachel E. Hile, Laura D. Hirshbein, Lisa Jacobson, Soraya Jenkins, Susie Keller, Jennifer Kelly, Carolyn Herbst Lewis, Alice O'Connor, Jess O'Keefe, Matthew A. Sutton, Karin Tamerius, and Warren Wood. Although some of you may argue with aspects of this book, I believe your comments and engagement have made the final book stronger than it otherwise would have been.

History relies on research, and I want to express my gratitude to those librarians and archivists who have helped me. Thank you to the friendly folks at the University of California at Santa Barbara's Davidson Library, especially the Interlibrary Loan staff, whose quickness, efficiency, and personal attention never failed to put a grateful smile on my face and obscure nineteenth-century texts into my possession. I also owe a great deal to the staff at the Helmke Library at Indiana University–Purdue University Fort Wayne, who went out of their way to find original documents when microfilm simply would not do. I also thank, too, the helpful archivists of the collections on which this book is based, including: the archives of the College of Physicians of Philadelphia; the Local History Room, Kalamazoo Public Library; Mount Holyoke College Archives and Special Collections; the Rare Book, Manuscript, and Special Collections at Duke University; History of Medicine Collection, Duke University Medical Center Library; Manuscripts and Archives, Yale University Library; Beinecke Rare Book and Manuscript Library, Yale University Library; Center for the History of Medicine, Francis A. Countway Library of Medicine, Harvard; Hagley Library and Museum; Special Collections, Lane Medical Library,

Stanford; The Bancroft Library, University of California at Berkeley; Special Collections, Davidson Library, University of California at Santa Barbara (UCSB).

Funding for this project has come from many generous sources, including: The IPFW Office of Research and External Support; The Purdue Research Foundation; the IPFW History Department; the UCSB History Department; the UCSB History Associates; the UCSB Graduate Division; the UCSB New Visions of Nature, Science, and Religion program; the University of California Humanities Research Institute (White Grant program); the University of California Interdisciplinary Psychoanalytic Consortium; the Philip and Aida Siff Educational Foundation; and the College of Physicians of Philadelphia.

I also want to thank those friends who were always willing to play the role of gracious host while I was on research trips, or who have provided much-needed emotional support while I worked on the book. *Teşekkür ederim* to Toshi Aono, Nicole Archambeau, Anne Barnhart, Shiva Barnhart, Michael Bender, Kim Bowers, Jason Bram, Renfield Bram, Jersey Joe Campo, Jessica Chapman, Andy Downs, Kathleen Duval, Alex Farr, Bob Frye, Josh Hoffman, Debrah Huffman, Justin Jennings, Michael Jerryson, Andy Jewett, Michelle Kern, Golem LeChat, Steven McKagan, Craig Ortsey, Anne Petersen, Lee Roberts, Mehran and Heather Sahami, John Sbardellati, Cathy Schuster, Michael Schuster, Joe Shanks, Tim Shanks, Aaron Small, Alec Small, Anya Small, Marty Smith, Jason Summers, Jamie Toole, Georgia Ulmschneider, Michael Wolf, and Karla Zepeda.

Most of all I want to thank my parents, John and Eleanor Schuster, to whom I dedicate this book.

Neurasthenic Nation

Introduction

Depression, irritability, insomnia, lethargy, indigestion, pain—these have long been part of what it means to be human. They have served to describe central characters in Shakespearean dramas, shaped our understanding of what it means to grow old, and defined some of the more unpleasant aspects of pregnancy. Considered for generations to be unfortunate but entirely normal aspects of life, by the turn of the twentieth century these conditions had begun to represent something new: the intolerable symptoms of illness.

It was the 1869 arrival of a disease known as *neurasthenia* that made Americans less accommodating of life's many mental and physical miseries. As the United States rushed toward industrial, technological, and social development, people worried that life had become too complicated, that the economy had become too turbulent, that domestic responsibilities had become too taxing, and that informational overload had created a fast-paced, modern society that sickened citizens. Physicians testified that the ill effects of modern life were indisputable and evidenced by an array of chronic symptoms, including depression, irritability, insomnia, lethargy, indigestion, a lack of ambition, an inability to concentrate, anxiety, headaches, muscle and joint pain, weight loss, impotence, amenorrhea, and both mental and physical collapse, any of which signified the potential presence of neurasthenia. In short, neurasthenia recast many unpleasant aspects of life as undesirable byproducts of a nation trying to evolve and improve faster than the natural abilities of its citizenry could keep pace.

This book suggests that America's experience with neurasthenia helped establish the quest for happiness and comfort as a fundamental aspect of modern American culture going into the twentieth century. Neurasthenia accomplished this by making discomfort and unhappiness seem like abnormal conditions—medical symptoms that required therapeutic treatment—and by establishing happiness and comfort as the norm of good health. This is not a story of professional medicine foisting its monolithic influence on an unsuspecting public; the medical profession during the late nineteenth century was much too disorganized, and too much lacked the authority, to do such a thing. Rather, the story of neurasthenia is one of reciprocity, wherein the medical profession, patients, and popular culture all interacted to help shape the disease in the imagination of one another. The constant interpretation, reinterpretation, and personalization of the condition and its many symptoms made for a vibrant exchange that essentially treated health, happiness, and comfort as commodities. Advertisers, thinkers, writers, reformers, and religious advocates, in addition to physicians and patients, all participated in this process by incorporating neurasthenia and its symptoms into economic, social, and cultural ventures that reinforced the notion that experiencing unhappiness and discomfort was the result of a sickness treatable through therapeutic purchases, social change, or spiritual conversion.

Neurasthenia was the characteristic illness of its day. The name derives from Greek and translates roughly to "lack of nerve energy." In the popular press, medical texts, and casual conversation, people often referred to the condition as *nervous prostration* or *nervous exhaustion,* and used venerable terms such as *nervousness* or simply *nerves* to describe the unhealthy enervation leading to the full-blown neurasthenic condition. The illness typically struck urbanites, especially those men and women carrying on busy lives stretched thin by responsibilities to their families, communities, and jobs. It was a chronic condition that might last anywhere from a few days to a few years before going dormant, always threatening to relapse.

What is more, Americans believed neurasthenia was absolutely new, a unique and admirable development in human history linked directly to their nation's struggle to improve itself and rise above other nations of the world. Although some neurasthenics were embarrassed by their condition, afraid that it might be interpreted as malingering or a lack of resolve, others took an element of martyred pride in their illness and saw it as evidence of hard work and of willingness to sacrifice personal health in the noble pursuit of excellence. Consequently, the illness possessed a social cachet that made it something to be talked about in public rather than whispered about in private. Comprehensive numbers of neurasthenia cases are impossible to calculate—it was a formal diagnosis often informally applied—but by the turn of the century the condition was ubiquitous and talk of it could be found throughout American households, popular literature, and commercial advertising. It achieved the rare distinction of becoming a fashionable illness, as famous personalities such as Jane Addams, Edith Wharton, and William James fell victim. It became, in the words of one physician, a "household word."[1]

Neurasthenia became a common diagnosis because it was an eminently versatile label, an umbrella term under which people included a myriad of symptoms and supposed causes. It covered ground comparable with a broad collection of twenty-first-century diagnoses, including bipolar disorder, clinical depression, chronic fatigue syndrome, fibromyalgia, post-traumatic stress disorder, anorexia nervosa, irritable bowel syndrome, migraines, environmental allergies (including hay fever), and a host of other chronic illnesses identified but not entirely cured by modern medicine.[2] Unlike tuberculosis, a well-known health threat from the time that consumed the lungs and other organs, neurasthenia lacked a clear physical pathology. Pioneers in the medical science of neurology imbued neurasthenia with a theoretical pathology, however, by describing the malady as a depletion of so-called nervous energy and resultant physical and mental exhaustion.

Produced by digestion and distributed through the body via the nervous system, nervous energy supposedly powered the body in much the same way electricity powered light bulbs and machinery and, just as an insufficient supply of electricity might cause bulbs to dim and machinery to malfunction, an insufficient supply of nervous energy might cause minds to dim and bodies to malfunction. The body-as-electrical-machine metaphor resonated within an American population fascinated with emerging technologies championed by people such as Thomas Edison and Alexander Graham Bell. It also helped explain why so many disparate symptoms, from headaches to impotence, could be traced back to the same medical condition. The neurasthenia diagnosis provided an elastic, protean concept of sickness that allowed Americans to better understand and speak about the nature of their mental and physical ailments.

Neurasthenia was a cultural as well as a medical construction, cobbled together from popular anxieties peculiar to the period, and spread along informational vectors. In expounding causes for the illness, early writers on neurasthenia directed suspicion toward the anxiety associated with modernization. Families left spacious countryside areas for burgeoning cities; men left the plow and field for the office and business; women left the parlor and family for the university and careers; speeding trains, rattling stock tickers, and clacking telegraphs created a fast-paced world: all these factors drained people of their nervous strength.

As the nineteenth century became the twentieth, groups outside the medical profession co-opted the idea of neurasthenia, wove it into their own literature, and greatly expanded the public discussion of the condition. Neurasthenia was cultural in nature and Americans understood the illness much differently than did Europeans, who had their own national versions of the disease. The American version also differed from that of the Chinese, who saw their traditional concepts of medicine reflected in a neurasthenia diagnosis that they continued to use well into the late twentieth century, long after mainstream American medicine set aside the label in favor of more physiologically and psychologically specific diagnoses.[3]

Neurasthenia was also a condition laden with economic implications. One of the central aspects of the disease was that it drained people's motivation and ability to work, so that, almost by definition, the sickness meant a loss of productivity. At the same time, the diagnosis gave people license to purchase and consume products and services that promised relief. In addition to doctors' bills, a neurasthenic could expect to pay for medical treatments ranging from relatively inexpensive electrotherapies to costly rest cures. A commercial economy developed around neurasthenia, with pharmaceutical companies, health resorts, self-help publishers, and even breakfast cereals each marketed as providing the best cure for modern nerves. The condition developed a reputation as a disease of the well-to-do, because it required money to embrace the diagnosis wholeheartedly and make wide use of treatments.

Neurasthenia ended up promoting lasting changes in American society as it helped people negotiate cultural tensions going into the twentieth century. Social conservatives sometimes employed the diagnosis to support their position that too much modern change was unhealthy, but others argued that poor health came from modern changes applied unevenly, a position that unleashed the potentially radical side of neurasthenia. As people witnessed changes around them in society, business, and technology, many became anxious that they were being left behind and were thus doomed to suffer unhappiness and discomfort for being premodern people in a modern world. Antiquated gender roles, a need for exercise, a want of inspiration—many diagnosed as neurasthenics saw these as lying at the root of their illness, evidence that they were having difficulty adapting to modern life. Therapy meant adopting more modern lifestyles or engaging in therapeutic activities such as taking mood-altering and pain-relieving medication, engaging in self-help spiritual movements, reconfiguring gender roles, going camping, and engaging in psychotherapy.

Readers today should beware of using a twenty-first-century eye to assess neurasthenia's integrity as an illness. Certainly there were malingerers who claimed to have been sick with neurasthenia to avoid work or responsibility—critics at the time made such accusations—but present research has not found enough examples to justify drawing the entire diagnosis into question. Also, observers today may suggest that neurasthenia was "all in the head," and consequently not an authentic disease. Neurasthenia experts at the turn of the twentieth century wrestled with this question, as well, and resolved the issue by recognizing that many physical symptoms had psychosomatic origins. Ultimately, trying to nail down what neurasthenia actually was or was not in a strictly medical sense threatens to remove the diagnosis from its historical context. The more important task is to identify how Americans from 1869 to 1920 perceived neurasthenia, and, overwhelmingly, they perceived neurasthenia and its symptoms to be a legitimate health concern.

By focusing on neurasthenia, this book largely bypasses discussion of a similar umbrella diagnosis of the period that shared many of neurasthenia's symptoms: hysteria. Identifying the differences between neurasthenia and hysteria is, and was, no easy task. After hearing that Harvard Medical School challenged its students to differentiate the two in an examination question, Dr. Morton Prince suggested in 1898 that drawing a sharp line between neurasthenia and hysteria was impossible. Nonetheless, physicians struggled to do so. Some doctors at the time believed hysteria developed out of severe neurasthenia. Others claimed that neurasthenia represented a variety of hysteria. Still more argued that neurasthenia and hysteria represented two independent conditions. Even famed neurologist S. Weir Mitchell decided to hedge diagnoses when he resubtitled his otherwise successful book *Fat and Blood* as "An Essay on the Treatment of Certain Forms of Neurasthenia and Hysteria." For much of the late nineteenth and early twentieth centuries, the two conditions were intertwined while the medical community struggled to define its diagnostic boundaries.[4]

Fortunately, the passage of time and the scholarship of many have highlighted qualitative aspects that help differentiate neurasthenia from hysteria. Neurasthenia possessed a certain American flavor, compared to hysteria's European quality, in large part because the United States stood at the center of neurasthenia research during the late nineteenth and early twentieth centuries while Europe led in studies on hysteria. Neurasthenia also allowed for more patient agency and nonmedical influence over the diagnosis than did hysteria; this occurred since the relative lack of professional authority possessed by American physicians in comparison with their European colleagues allowed neurasthenia to develop via a reciprocal cycle of information between American physicians, patients, and popular culture. Reciprocity, and the patient agency it entailed, also allowed neurasthenia to develop an aura of distinction that hysteria lacked. Finally, contemporary understandings of neurasthenia and hysteria are influenced by the fact that neurasthenia quickly disappeared in American after 1920. Hysteria, however, continued to occupy a place within American culture, thanks largely to the twentieth-century popularity of Freud and his European studies on the topic. Neurasthenia is a dated, unfamiliar concept to most people alive in the twenty-first century, while hysteria has continued to exert a familiar, if perhaps ahistorical, influence over the ways people speak about health and behavior.[5]

Neurasthenic Nation examines the story of neurasthenia and the reciprocal relationships the condition helped create among physicians, patients, and popular culture. With the first articles published on neurasthenia in 1869 came a period of familiarization between America's medical profession and the public in which physicians figured out how to integrate their services for treating unhappiness and discomfort into the lives of the nation's growing urban population. Neurasthenia's expansion of the medical market did not go unnoticed by business persons and journalists, who employed the diagnosis to lucratively advertise medical contraptions and medicines and provide grist for news and feature stories. By the 1890s, the reciprocal cycle of information about neurasthenia had made the condition a force in popular culture that influenced people's spirituality, their concepts of gender, and their lifestyles and leisure activities. After the turn of the twentieth century, changes in American medicine, and progressive laws governing advertising, began to disrupt the reciprocal exchange of information upon which neurasthenia thrived, however, so that by 1920 the once ubiquitous diagnosis had run its course and was rapidly losing medical and cultural relevance.

In a larger sense, the story of neurasthenia is indicative of Americans' struggle to create a more perfect union through the pursuit of health, happiness, and comfort. The intolerance of unhappiness and discomfort associated with neurasthenia, and the expectation that good health could be attained through therapeutic activities and purchases, left an indelible impression on the United States that has continued to exist long after the neurasthenia diagnosis faded into academic obscurity.

Chapter 1

Professional Medicine and the Discovery of Neurasthenia

In front of an auditorium filled with his medical colleagues of the Boston Society for Medical Improvement, Harvard neurologist James Jackson Putnam began his 1895 address by noting "There is hardly a subject in practical medicine which is of wider interest than the study of . . . neurasthenia." Putnam was not alone in recognizing the importance of the neurasthenia diagnosis to the American medical profession, as Cornell's Charles Dana later characterized neurasthenia to the Boston Society of Psychiatry and Neurology as "our one great national malady" and a "distinctive and precious pathological possession."[1] When the neurasthenia diagnosis made its debut in 1869, few people could have predicted that it would become such a favorite of the American medical community. After all, it lacked a clear pathology or physical cause, and its symptoms varied widely. Yet the two doctors who both published on neurasthenia in 1869 without apparent knowledge of the other—Edwin H. Van Deusen in the *American Journal of Insanity,* and George M. Beard in the *Boston Medical and Surgical Journal*—each suspected that he had discovered an important new disease.[2]

Van Deusen was technically the first to publish on neurasthenia, yet it was Beard and another physician, S. Weir Mitchell, who had the largest impact on framing the diagnosis. One reason for Van Deusen's lack of influence traces back to his profession as an alienist, the nineteenth-century title given to psychiatrists working in asylums and commissioned with caring for those who were insane and *alienated* from the rest of society. As the superintendent of the Michigan State Asylum at Kalamazoo, Van Deusen represented a branch of medicine seen by the public and other physicians during the late nineteenth century as dated and out of touch with America's mainstream medical needs. Beard, on the other hand, was a neurologist and part of a new breed of medical specialists who positioned themselves as alternatives to alienists and asylum care. He crafted neurasthenia into a disease of high civilization, a result of a modern society that pushed people too hard, causing them to become sick with mental and physical symptoms. This was not insanity, Beard stressed, merely exhaustion. After Beard's death in 1883, Mitchell, also a neurologist, became the foremost authority on neurasthenia. Mitchell helped cultivate a sense of exclusivity around the disease while recognizing its considerable emotional dimensions, which warranted lucrative, physician-guided therapies that ultimately helped fuel the turn-of-the-century professionalization of medicine.

The story of neurasthenia and the practices of Van Deusen, Beard, and Mitchell illustrate the reciprocity that the neurasthenia diagnosis helped create between sick Americans and the medical profession during the late nineteenth century. Van Deusen's work on neurasthenia landed flat because it could not overcome professional and public suspicion of the asylum care he advocated. Conversely, Beard and Mitchell were able to broaden the appeal of neurasthenia and cultivate a therapeutic rapport with Americans. They did so by creating explanations of, and treatments for, the condition that reflected their clientele's nationalistic, class, and racial sensibilities. Patients benefited because the neurasthenia diagnosis legitimated their mental, emotional, and physical ailments and allowed for sympathy and care. Physicians also benefited, especially those in the emerging specialty of neurology, because neurasthenia cultivated a large body of middle- and upper-class patients who legitimated the role of doctors as caretakers of the nation's happiness and comfort and helped financed the building of the medical profession at the start of the twentieth century.[3]

Edwin H. Van Deusen (1828–1909)

In Kalamazoo, Michigan, Dr. Edwin Holmes Van Deusen was a celebrity. He oversaw the construction of the town's asylum and served as its superintendent for twenty years. A devoted member of St. Luke's Episcopal Church, he was a community benefactor who, with his wife Cynthia, contributed tens of thousands of dollars to his local congregation, hospital, and library. In his obituary, the *Kalamazoo Gazette* proclaimed that Dr. Van Deusen "will always be regarded as the greatest philanthropist of Kalamazoo County."[4] Ironically, the things that made Van Deusen a great man in Kalamazoo—his leadership at the asylum and his dedication to the largely rural community—also made him a weak spokesperson for the neurasthenia diagnosis.

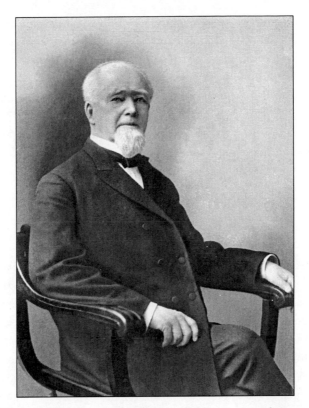

Figure 1   Edwin H. Van Deusen. An alienist, Van Deusen was the superintendent of the Michigan Asylum for the Insane at Kalamazoo from 1859 to 1878, and the first to publish an essay on neurasthenia, in 1869.

From David Fisher and Frank Little, *Compendium of History and Biography of Kalamazoo County, Michigan* [Chicago: A. W. Bowen and Co., 1906], 116. Image courtesy of the Kalamazoo Public Library, Local History Room.

Van Deusen was born on August 29, 1828, in Livingston, New York, into a successful merchant and milling family.[5] He excelled at academics and, after attending local schools and taking preparatory courses at Claverack Academy, he entered Williams College, where he earned his bachelor of arts and master's degrees. Between degrees, he took classes at the College of Physicians and Surgeons of New York City, where he graduated with distinction, and received an internship at the New York Hospital in 1850. While in New York, Van Deusen volunteered with fellow interns to battle a typhus epidemic that ended up decimating medical personnel, leaving him one of the last surviving hospital physicians. The dedication and ability he showed during this epidemic earned him a reputation as one of New York's up-and-coming medical talents, and soon he attracted the attention of Dr. John P. Gray, the young and ambitious superintendent of the Utica State Lunatic Asylum, who saw administrative potential in Van Deusen and hired him as an assistant in 1853, thereby giving him his start as an alienist. Within a few years, Gray had accepted a job as superintendent of the asylum being built in Kalamazoo, but second thoughts about the move made him rescind his acceptance and kept him in the New York asylum system. As Gray's protégé, Van Deusen assumed responsibility for overseeing the opening and operations of the Kalamazoo Asylum; by 1858, he had moved from upstate New York to Michigan to begin his new job as asylum superintendent.

Van Deusen's article on neurasthenia grew from his attempt to explain what he thought was Kalamazoo's unusually high proportion of female patients. In an article, "Observations on a Form of Nervous Prostration, (Neurasthenia,) Culminating in Insanity," Van Deusen suggested that the answer lay with Michigan's status as a pioneer state. Unlike families in the relatively urban east coast, families in Michigan tended to live on isolated farms. Although the jobs involved in farming were enough to keep men busy Van Deusen believed, the lives of farm women, especially those with small children, were "exhausting and depressing to a degree of which but a few [persons not farm wives] are likely to form any correct conception." Usually marrying young, a new farm wife could expect to be transferred "from a home in which she had enjoyed a requisite measure of social and intellectual recreation" to "an isolated farmhouse . . . [and be] subject to a daily routine of very monotonous household labor." Husbands were of little help, Van Deusen remarked, as they usually came home exhausted from their own day's work, ate, and went to sleep early, leaving wives "to pass the long and lonely evening with [their] needle[s]" and without adequate companionship.[6] Separated from their friends and family and constantly occupied with mindless chores, farm wives would dwell on their predicament and be unable to wrest their minds away from their plight of isolation. Neurasthenia was the all too common result, Van Deusen explained, as farm wives slipped into a general malaise, which in turn led to impaired digestion, physical weakening, and admission into the Kalamazoo Asylum.

Although Van Deusen identified farm wives as particularly prone to neurasthenia, he believed men and students also suffered from anxiety that could lead to the disease. For their part, men were threatened by "great responsibility" at work, which made "heavy demands upon the nervous energies of the individual." If isolation served as the catalyst for neurasthenia among farm wives, then the possibility of financial failure led to neurasthenia among men. With a man expected to be the family provider, his economic shortcomings represented a "pecuniary embarrassment" that might cause poor sleep and improper eating habits, which could grow into neurasthenic despondency. Making matters worse, according to Van Deusen, was the "rash, restless, speculative character" of American business, which generated economic instability that could catch entire communities in a web of anxiety. Schools and the "hothouse" educational system that pressured young men and women to exceed their natural intellectual talents also led to neurasthenia by creating anxiety among students. Whether neurasthenia struck women, men, adults, or children, Van Deusen believed a fundamental aspect of the disease was "mental alienation" that caused patients to become absorbed with their own invalidism and emotionally isolated from others.[7]

Neurasthenic symptoms listed by Van Deusen included an array of mental, physical, and emotional markers that would eventually become standard in descriptions of the disease. Depression, mania, anxiety, irritability, impaired intellect, indigestion, malnourishment, insomnia, physical weakness, and neuralgia were all possible signs of neurasthenia, and, due to heightened excitability, neurasthenics were highly vulnerable to the effects of alcohol and also easily embarrassed. Neurasthenics shared a profound distrust of things in which they previously had had faith: the highly religious doubted God and the church; those who aspired to material wealth dreaded inevitable poverty; those dedicated to their spouses became consumed with jealousy. Such behavior only worked to increase anxiety and make neurasthenia worse. Van Deusen's description of the disease, so similar to the symptomatology that would later characterize the standard understanding of neurasthenia proffered by Beard and Mitchell, differed in one key respect: prognosis. Although most people by 1900 considered neurasthenia a chronic, but nonfatal illness, Van Deusen argued that the condition could snowball out of control and deteriorate to the point of insanity, coma, and death.[8]

Luckily for neurasthenics, Van Deusen believed if the condition were detected and treated early enough it could be cured without threat of relapse. Treatments included prescribing a nutritious diet, administering nerve tonics (popular ones of the day were quinine, arsenic, strychnine, iron, and phosphorus), providing the occasional morphine shot to alleviate insomnia, and giving soothing sponge baths to calm emotions and quell pain. In difficult cases, a physician might advise a patient to change jobs to escape occupational anxieties. Van Deusen also suggested "moral treatment" such as adopting a recreational activity designed to provide gentle exercise and occupy the mind so that it did not dwell on invalidism. Traveling was of dubious value, he thought, because, while a change in scene might seem the perfect cure for those sick and tired with their lives, the hassle that often accompanied traveling might cause more harm than good. As an asylum superintendent, Van Deusen predicated treatments on the opportunity for inpatient care that allowed "careful daily observation at the bedside" and prescription adjustments with each new symptom. He proudly declared that, so long as institutional care was available, he found neurasthenics' "improvement, both mental and physical, has been *pari passu*, and in no case has there been a return of the disease."[9] Ideally, neurasthenics were temporary patients, people who visited asylums for treatment and advice in much the same way those with physical injuries might visit hospitals for aid in their recovery. Neurasthenics, after all, were not yet insane and did not need to be locked up; rather, they were injured and in need of the healing that, Van Deusen believed, asylums were in the best position to offer.

By the 1870s, however, asylums did not carry the therapeutic cachet they had possessed decades earlier. During the first part of the nineteenth century, asylums arose in America as a humane and reportedly effective way of treating mental illness. Innovations by Europeans such as Philippe Pinel and William Tuke led to the development of moral therapy, a treatment strategy that rejected prison cells, corporal punishment, and harsh restraints, and replaced them with structured regimes of exercise, church attendance, and daily work; the belief was that if the mentally unstable could carry on (dress, act, eat, and amuse themselves) according to basic social norms, then sanity would eventually develop. In response to campaigns by American reformers such as Dorothea Dix and the remarkable (if outlandish) cure rates initially claimed by early asylums (the Hartford Retreat for the Insane listed a 91 percent cure rate in 1827, for instance, and both the Eastern Lunatic Asylum and the Ohio Lunatic Asylum claimed a less modest 100 percent cure rate in 1843), states began, in the 1830s, funding the construction and operation of public asylums. Within a few generations, however, it had become clear that the heady optimism that led to building asylums in the United States was misplaced. Faced with what were in reality dismal cure rates, consumed with administrative duties, and responsible for overcrowded facilities, alienists of the second half of the nineteenth century found their credibility eroded as they gained the notorious reputation of being little more than jailers guarding the asylum gates.[10]

Nineteenth-century writers and reporters stoked the public's mistrust of asylums with a rash of unsettling stories depicting nightmarish conditions, false imprisonments, and sadistic therapies. Edgar Allen Poe's short story "The System of Dr. Tarr and Prof. Fether" (1845), for instance, provided a carnivalesque scenario in which the patients were, quite literally, running the asylum.

On a much darker note, Isaac Hunt's *Three Years in a Mad-House* (1851) gave a deeply disturbing account of the author's dreadful experience trapped as a patient inside the Maine Hospital for the Insane. "What a benevolent brotherhood!" Hunt sarcastically exclaimed. "How kind is the State to build a human slaughter house, for physicians to torture and murder human beings in! What benevolent hospitality!" Nellie Bly, the pen name of twenty-three-year-old investigative reporter Elizabeth Jane Cochran, went undercover and masqueraded as a madwoman to experience asylum life in 1887 for a series of articles published in Joseph Pulitzer's *New York World* and compiled later that year as *Ten Days in a Mad-House*. Bly's experience was distinctly unpleasant. "The insane asylum on Blackwell's Island is a human rat-trap," she ominously informed her readers. "It is easy to get in, but once there it is impossible to get out."[11] If having neurasthenia meant being treated in places like these, most Americans would have resisted the diagnosis.

Van Deusen himself became embroiled in a sordid tale of false imprisonment and cruel asylum treatment. While visiting her daughter in Michigan during the summer of 1874, Nancy J. Newcomer, a Toledo physician, fell ill with anemia and "nervous exhaustion"—a synonym for neurasthenia—and became highly agitated. Her son-in-law contacted the local superintendent in charge of the poor, who had Newcomer whisked away to Van Deusen's asylum, where she was committed as an "insane pauper" and held against her will from October 1874 until her release in August 1875. After her release, Newcomer filed a lawsuit against Van Deusen and his asylum for false imprisonment, thus setting in motion a legal case that eventually found its way to the Supreme Court of Michigan.[12]

According to court records, the prosecution played on the public's mistrust and fear of asylums by portraying Van Deusen as a "keeper of a great prison in which he made it his business to entrap and confine weak and helpless people." Attorneys successfully convinced the jury that Van Deusen "stood at the door of this hideous place of confinement ready to seize and thrust into its hopeless cells every victim who avarice or malignity might entice or drag into his reach." Newcomer claimed to have been forced to bathe in soiled water, to undergo physical abuse, and never to have been taken seriously by the staff; her own credentials as a physician meant nothing when others thought she was mad. Van Deusen was eager, the prosecution argued, to strike a nefarious deal with Newcomer's son-in-law to commit her so that the son-in-law could inherit her property. The jury in the initial trial found Van Deusen guilty and ordered him to pay damages of $6,000. On appeal, in 1879 the Michigan Supreme Court reversed this decision and ended up issuing an

opinion, written by Justice Thomas M. Cooley, apologizing for the unfair treatment given Van Deusen in the first trial. Despite the eventual verdict of not
guilty, the trial took its toll on Van Deusen, and he retired from his position at
Kalamazoo in 1878, citing overwork and poor health. The appeals trial, *Van
Deusen v. Newcomer* (1879), set an important precedent for alienists and asylum care: so long as asylum superintendents acted in good faith, they could
not be held liable for mistakenly committing a sane person.[13] Good faith or
not, the trial underscores America's suspicion of alienists (and all things
"insane") during the late nineteenth century.

Given this suspicion and mistrust surrounding alienists, it is hardly surprising that by the 1870s they were embroiled in a professional battle with
neurologists, a relatively new breed of specialists who thought alienists stood
in the way of scientific progress and access to patients. Neurologists represented a younger generation of physicians who had made a name for themselves during the Civil War treating soldiers suffering from gunshot wounds
and other battlefield injuries. Physiology was extremely important for neurologists, who traced mental and physical disorders back to disruptions in the
nervous system. Scientific was their word for their physiological approach to
medicine, which combined empirical observation with laboratory experimentation. Conflicts between alienists and neurologists centered on who could
legitimately lay claim to being most knowledgeable on issues concerning
mental health. For most of the nineteenth century, alienists were in a superior
position, as they controlled the asylums and consequently had a lock on
America's collection of mental health patients. In 1878, the same year Van
Deusen appealed his conviction for false imprisonment to the Michigan
Supreme Court, New York neurologists led by Dr. Edward Spitzka called for
an investigation of that state's asylum system, run by Van Deusen's former
mentor, Dr. John P. Gray. Spitzka's goal was to loosen alienists' tight grip on
the asylum population, as well as to gain access to patients, and his often
vitriolic attacks (he famously called Gray "an indifferent, superficial man,
owing his position merely to political buffoonery") only served to deepen the
divisions between neurologists and alienists.[14]

The professional rivalry between the two professions publicly erupted in
spectacular fashion with the trial of President James Garfield's assassin, Charles
Guiteau; this was a media event that dominated the nation's headlines from
autumn 1881 until summer 1882. By all accounts, Guiteau was an eccentric
man, but whether or not he was insane, and therefore unfit to be hanged, was
another question entirely. Alienists, led by Gray, sided with the prosecution's
contention that Guiteau was sane, and gave copious testimony regarding the

meaning of insanity. Neurologists, led by Spitzka, were employed by the defense to prove Guiteau's insanity. It was a public showdown with professional legitimacy on the line, and when the jury found Guiteau guilty, sane, and deserving of hanging, indignant neurologists pronounced the trial a national embarrassment. Proclaiming the Guiteau case tantamount to a witch hunt, neurologist George M. Beard denounced the opinion of alienists and the court: "Washington has taken its place side by side with the trials of Salem, in the permanent record of judicial cruelty and non-expertness."[15] The Guiteau trial was a pyrrhic victory for alienists, for, though they convinced a jury to find a presidential assassin competent and guilty, they did little to convince the rest of the American medical community to see them as still on the cutting edge of mental health research.

Van Deusen did not have a lasting effect on the development of the neurasthenia diagnosis because his association with asylum care placed him out of step with the public and much of the medical profession. The very title of Van Deusen's article, as well as the journal that published it (the *American Journal of Insanity*) provided a direct link between neurasthenia and insanity that would have made patients and physicians alike shy away from such a diagnosis. Other factors of Van Deusen's diagnosis also mitigated his influence, such as its emphasis on lonely farm wives rather than on middle-class urban women (the latter proving to have the growing numbers and wealth to provide a reliable clientele), and the doctor's own Kalamazoo location far from traditional centers of medical influence such as Philadelphia, Boston, and New York. Thus it came down to neurologist Beard's description of neurasthenia to provide the foundation upon which neurasthenia grew into one of the most influential diagnoses of its time and, in the words of historian Charles Rosenberg, guaranteed Beard "a small, but apparently secure place in the accepted canon of medical history."[16]

George Miller Beard (1839–1883)

Beard was a man of many interests who reveled in public debates over the meaning of science and ambitiously sought to combine health and modernization into a grand theory of medical sociology. He may not have been particularly brilliant, but he was an engaged member of East Coast urban life (his home was in New York City) and had a knack for synthesizing ideas and developments happening around him. Beard published his first article on neurasthenia at the end of April 1869 in the *Boston Medical and Surgical Journal,* then set major work on neurasthenia to the side for over a decade as he dedicated himself to numerous other projects, including writing essays on spiritualism,

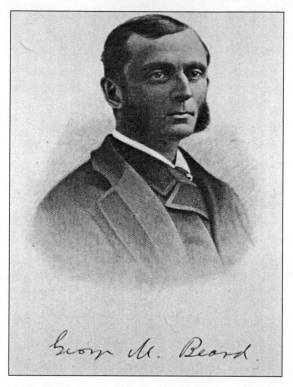

Figure 2   George M. Beard. A New York City neurologist, Beard helped make neurasthenia one of the most common diagnoses of the late nineteenth century, and his 1881 book, *American Nervousness,* stood as the most authoritative text on the disease.

Photo courtesy of the National Library of Medicine, History of Medicine collection.

electricity, temperance, aging, skin disease, tumors, and phobias. He returned to neurasthenia with two books, *A Practical Treatise on Nervous Exhaustion (Neurasthenia)* (1880) and his magnum opus, *American Nervousness: Its Causes and Consequences* (1881).[17] Beard's influence on neurasthenia developed because he successfully cultivated a public image as a dedicated man of science, and created a narrative for the disease that made the diagnosis relevant for a late nineteenth-century population going through profound social and cultural changes associated with modernization.

Beard, the youngest of four children, was born on May 8, 1839, in Montville, Connecticut. His father, Reverend S. F. Beard, and brothers were Congregationalist ministers. After attending Philips Academy in Andover, Massachusetts, Beard spent two years teaching before entering Yale University in 1858. At Yale, he was a gregarious student who excelled in debate and writing, edited the *Yale Literary Magazine*, and developed a powerful fascination with science. Graduating in 1862, he spent a year at the Yale School of Medicine, and in the fall of 1863 he traveled to New York, where he took classes at the regional College of Physician and Surgeons. Less than a year later, he found himself part of the Union war effort as an acting assistant surgeon for the U.S. Navy, a post he held for eighteen months, resigning in 1865. He returned to his medical studies in New York, and in 1866 earned his M.D. with an emphasis in neurology from the College of Physicians and Surgeons.[18]

Although Beard did not follow his many American colleagues to Europe to finish his education, after graduation he began a rigorous professional life informed by European experimental science. He bought the large practice of another doctor and formed a partnership with Alphonso D. Rockwell, an associate with whom he built a career in electrotherapeutics. The medical science of neurology was in its infancy during this time, and neurologists struggled to define themselves vis-à-vis other branches of medicine such as psychiatry, gynecology, and general practice. For Beard, this meant combining physiology with the scientific work of others, especially Germans such as Emil du Bois-Reymond (1818–1896), who experimented on the electrical nature of nerve impulses, and Julius Robert von Mayer (1814–1878) and Hermann von Helmholtz (1821–1894), both of whom worked on thermodynamics.[19] He developed a general theory of health rooted in the supposed existence of vital biological energy that ran through the nervous system in much the same way electricity ran through copper wiring. Just as electricity powered motors and gadgets, so too did biological nervous energy power the body's organs, muscles, and brain. Problems arose and neurasthenia occurred, Beard contended, when an individual's supply of nervous energy ran low, causing his or her body to malfunction. To counteract the body's loss of energy, he and Rockwell pioneered the use of mild electrotherapy, a procedure that was at first received dubiously by the medical community, but that became a commonplace treatment in the late nineteenth century, thanks in part to Beard and Rockwell's publishing efforts.[20]

Beard had an almost fetishistic fascination with science. He was never particularly religious, and, although family members thought of him as Christian, his professional and personal friends knew him as agnostic. Science took the place of religion for him, as it provided a philosophical lens through which he understood the world. What exactly he envisioned science to be is not altogether clear (he used the term without much explanation), but his published work and private correspondence reveal the rough parameters of his scientific approach. He appreciated midcentury experimental science, especially that coming out of Germany. His own work would, by today's standards, largely be considered social science, as it tended to focus on people's behavior and depend on the validity of human testimony rather than investigate the hidden physical world as revealed by microscopes or chemical reactions. One of his rare ventures into the laboratory was in partnership with Thomas Edison, whom he greatly respected and with whom he claimed to have identified a "newly discovered force" that he described with sweeping theory that today might be considered similar to an explanation of radio waves.

For scientific logic, Beard relied heavily on Baconian induction, and he would compile long lists of evidence, which he scanned in search of patterns and relationships. His M.D. thesis, "Longevity of Brain Workers," for instance, identified the occupations and ages of scores of thinkers and artists throughout history, from which he concluded that smart people lived an unusually long time. As to whether the ability to think great thoughts was inherited, Beard simply opened an encyclopedia of American biographies and recorded three hundred names at random; upon seeing that over two hundred of the names were related in some way, he concluded that the ability to think great thoughts was indeed an inherited characteristic.[21] He aimed his analysis toward dramatic, generalized conclusions and did not concern himself overly with alternative perspectives, causal subtleties, or exceptions. When it came to scientific theory, he was hardly an innovator.

Beard was confident that science could explain all phenomena if given enough information. In bestowing ultimate explanatory power to the process of science, Beard followed what some have called a "religion of science," wherein he and others saw science, especially empiricism imported from Europe, as the key to identifying Truth. For Beard and his science-minded colleagues, this meant being able to differentiate credible practitioners of science from mere quacks who might sully its reputation by spreading misinformation. The time had come, Beard told readers of *Appletons' Journal* in 1869, for "scientific research" to rid society of the superstition and delusion caused by "political or social prejudice" (a somewhat ironic statement, as Beard also suggested that science proved blacks were inferior to whites in "mental and moral character").[22] Science could not rid the world of false ideas by itself, however, and Beard believed it took messengers—experts like himself—to spread knowledge to the masses.

Beard furthered his public reputation as a committed scientist and public intellectual in the 1870s by waging a campaign against spiritualism. Spiritualism, the belief that spirits of the dead could interact with the world of the living, began growing in America in the 1850s as newspapers started publicizing the exploits and séances of mediums, who claimed to be able to communicate with the afterlife. By the 1870s, spiritualism had entered America's mainstream, and in 1875 advocates founded the Theosophical Society to further spiritualist investigation and provide a clearinghouse of information on the movement. Indeed, a list of those who engaged in spiritualism includes some of the most respected names in nineteenth-century society and culture, including Harriet Beecher Stowe, William Lloyd Garrison, Horace Greeley, Mary Todd Lincoln, Benjamin Wade, Lydia Maria Child, William Cullen Bryant, James Fenimore Cooper, and William James.[23]

Beard's campaign against spiritualism rested on the premise that a physical explanation could be found for what spiritualists claimed were supernatural events. In October 1874 he visited Chittenden, Vermont, to observe the spiritual work of Horatio and William Eddy, better known as the Eddy Brothers. Hosting séances in which spirits reportedly played music, threw objects, signed cards, and materialized for people to see and feel, the Eddys had risen to fame a few months earlier when Col. Henry Steel Olcott, a respected Civil War veteran and New York lawyer, began closely studying the brothers and concluded that they were in fact authentic mediums who could establish contact with spirits. Olcott soon published his findings in a book titled *People from the Other World* (1875).[24] For his 1874 visit, arriving incognito and acting the part of a disheveled simpleton, Beard participated in a séance with the brothers and collected data to debunk their claim to supernatural spiritual contact. In an editorial for New York's *Daily Graphic*, Beard claimed that his "scientific observation" proved that the Eddys were skilled contortionists who, in the dim light of the séance, could "pass themselves off as dwarfs or, by the addition of a high head dress and a little stretching, might personate a giant." This, combined with a "benumbing arm trick," created the impression of supernatural intervention that, he said, would fool most people but not the trained eye of a scientist such as himself.[25]

Beard investigated neurasthenia with the same aplomb with which he sought to disprove spiritualism. Although there is no evidence that he ever met Van Deusen or read his work, his depiction of neurasthenia was remarkably similar to Van Deusen's. Both claimed that the condition represented an impoverishment of nervous energy (as the name implies) caused by unhappy or anxiety-ridden lives. Both suggested that excessive brain work and fixated thoughts were risk factors. Both listed similar symptoms, including neuralgia, lethargy, insomnia, anxiety, and depression. Both prescribed the therapeutic use of a proper diet, rest, mild exercise, fresh air, and tonics of strychnine, phosphorus, iron, and arsenic. A major difference between the two men's versions of neurasthenia came down to context, with Beard's presentation resonating with the new generation of Americans growing in power and influence in the last part of the nineteenth century. Publication of Beard's work in both professional journals such as the *Boston Medical and Surgical Journal* (the precursor to today's *New England Journal of Medicine*) and more popular texts such as *American Nervousness* reflect the broad appeal of his ideas.

The effectiveness and influence of Beard's explanation of neurasthenia stemmed from his linking the diagnosis to everyday aspects of American lives. Tooth decay, baldness, the "finely cut" beauty of American women, America's love for "grotesque and exaggerated" humor, Americans' gift for oratory, and the American tendency to shorten words were all the products of Americans' excessive use of nervous energy, he argued in *American Nervousness*. Five things, he claimed, distinctly set modern America apart from past civilizations: steam power, the periodical press, the telegraph, the sciences, and the "mental activity of women."[26] These were generally good developments, in his opinion, but they contributed to an inhospitable environment that overtaxed citizens' nervous energy and prevented proper rest and recuperation. Steam power, for instance, led to industrialization and faster transportation, but also resulted in regimented working conditions. Modern women had more options to cultivate their minds and follow artistic pursuits than ever before, but lack of physical labor made them more delicate, and the pressure to keep up with newly educated peers increased anxiety. Beard pointed to other issues as well: the proliferation of clocks and watches may have helped Americans become more prompt and efficient, but it also created the constant fear of being late; the spread of trolleys, omnibuses, and railroads signaled growth and investment, but their unrhythmic rattling and clacking frayed nerves and reminded people they were far from the soothing rumble of nature's waterfalls. Neurasthenia, in a sense, was a growing pain of American modernization and represented "part of the compensation for our [nation's] progress and refinement."[27]

The hardest-hit citizens, Beard argued, were the brain workers who toiled in a modern age of regularly changing information. Van Deusen had also written of the threat from brain work, but it was Beard who framed such work as a common characteristic of modern life. The telegraph and the daily press bombarded people constantly with new events so that even breakfast was made hectic by the morning newspaper's report of a distant train wreck or an upcoming election. Thomas Edison alone kept capitalists in suspense and distressed, with his inventions, according to Beard. Business had become a national, even international, endeavor, and the modern fascination with the stock market, for which Edison's stock ticker was at least partially responsible, had multiplied anxieties that were further intensified by the habit of buying on the margin and by the prevalent "boom or bust" mentality. In a statement more forceful than that made by Van Deusen, Beard argued that the volatile economy even trickled down to the family level, causing domestic and financial troubles as well as spreading a pervasive sense of uncertainty about the future. American liberty itself became a cause of modern nervousness, as citizens struggled to better themselves, influence politics, and wrestle with religious issues. Three questions weighed heavily on the modern American mind, Beard posited: "How shall we keep from starving? Who is to be the next President? And where shall we go when we die?"[28] Neurasthenia did not simply denote the presence of sickness; Beard argued it indicated the presence of an active mind, a competitive character, a lover of liberty—in short, the quintessential American. It is hardly surprising that Beard nicknamed neurasthenia "American nervousness" and that Europeans sometimes, usually with derision, called it the "American disease."

Beard infused his discussion of neurasthenia with a powerful nationalist sentiment that supported the idea that America was an exceptional country in the history of nations: "All this is modern, and originally American; and no age, no country, and no form of civilization, not Greece, nor Rome, nor Spain, nor the Netherlands, in the days of their glory, possessed such maladies," he explained to readers. Beard believed in evolution, and positioned himself as the American counterpart to Herbert Spencer, the British sociologist and champion of social Darwinism. In an article published in 1883, shortly before his death, Beard remarked how Spencer's sociological work closely paralleled his own work on neurasthenia, even going so far as to suggest that Spencer might have co-opted his ideas. Neurasthenia was *American* nervousness, Beard told his readers, and the disease stood as proof that their nation had evolved beyond the rest of the world. While the citizens of presumably less modern nations, including European states, still suffered from classic illnesses such as gout, rheumatism, and fever, neurasthenia, Beard claimed, represented the next evolutionary stage in illness, a disease that, as strange as it might sound, actually helped protect its victims from other diseases, such as fevers, which, he believed, were lower on the evolutionary tree. "If Gambetta had been a nervous man—a brain-bankrupt—he would probably have survived his wound," Beard suggested of the French republican leader accidentally killed when a revolver misfired on New Year's Eve of 1882–1883.[29] Neurasthenics, despite chronic discomfort and languishing, were longer-lived and, in their own way, hardier than non-neurasthenics.

Growing from his belief that neurasthenia was primarily an illness of civilization and modern liberty, Beard's description of the disease was rife

with religious, racial, and regional assumptions. Catholics were relatively safe
from neurasthenia because their church made important theological decisions,
thereby relieving members of the "burden of religion" that caused Protestants
to be nervous. Southern whites generally avoided the disease because, whereas
"a Northerner worships the new, the Southerner [worships] the old," thereby
avoiding the burden of nerve-wracking innovation. American Indians were
supposedly safe from neurasthenia because they did not overtax their mental
capacities and were content to live in ignorance and with an "utter want of
curiosity"; in addition, Beard believed their uncivilized, physical lives spent
mostly outdoors made for incredibly robust men and women who were rarely
made sick by any illness. Like Indians, American blacks, especially in the
south, supposedly lived primitive, hardy lives and possessed "immature
minds" indifferent to "nature's mysteries" and, unlike civilized whites, lived
"not for science or ideas, but for the senses and emotions."[30] By explaining who
was not susceptible to neurasthenia—Catholics, southerners, Indians, blacks—
Beard was framing neurasthenia as primarily a white, Anglo-Saxon, Protestant,
Yankee condition. In so doing, he, and by extension neurasthenia, co-opted and
moved forward the socially exclusive belief that northern, white, Protestant
society stood at the center of American life and civilization, an idea that would
gain weight in succeeding decades as new immigrants arrived in greater numbers from the Mediterranean and eastern Europe. If neurasthenics were the
quintessential Americans, then northern, white Protestants were the quintessential neurasthenics.

Ambitious as always, Beard cast a wide net with neurasthenia and sought
to make it, and the doctors who treated it, part of a larger movement developing in the social sciences. "The philosophic study of the several branches of
sociology, politics, charities, history, [and] education," Beard claimed in his
preface to *American Nervousness*, "shall never be even in the direction of scientific precision or completeness until it shall have absorbed some, at least, of
the suggestions of this problem of American Nervousness." Indeed, "to solve it
in all its interlacings, to unfold its marvelous phenomena and trace them back
to their sources and forward to their future developments, is to solve the problem of sociology itself," he explained with optimistic wonder.[31] The late nineteenth century was an exciting time for followers of science, who believed that,
given the proper research and experimental models, nearly any problem could
be conquered, including the economic instability, poverty, and crime prevalent
in the United States. Cities became laboratories as social scientists sought to
join their colleagues in the physical, chemical, and biological sciences by using
empirical and experimental approaches to better understand the world.[32]

Through the neurasthenia diagnosis, Beard sought to add citizens' health to the mix of concerns addressed by scientifically minded urban reformers.

With neurasthenia, Beard positioned physicians as the immediate solution to the enervating influence of modern American life. Asylums were not part of the picture, nor were the so-called heroic procedures that were common in the first half of the nineteenth century, a period that saw induced bleeding, vomiting, diarrhea, and blistering as proper treatment. As one might expect (considering the nature of his practice with Rockwell), Beard emphasized the therapeutic virtues of electrotherapy, which he claimed was the most direct way of recharging the body's energy supply. Such treatment was a relatively easy procedure, requiring only a galvanized or faradic battery and an anode and cathode. Beard's use of electricity was a mild electric current applied to sore areas and the scalp that might cause minor twitching or feel like a gentle massage (it is akin to what is today known as Transcutaneous Electrical Nerve Stimulation, or TENS). The effect soothed patients, relieved soreness, and gave the impression that their bodies were literally being replenished with vitalizing energy.

By many accounts, Beard's electrotherapy worked well and patients left sessions feeling refreshed and invigorated. As to why it worked, Beard claimed to fellow physicians—not to the public or within any of his popularly available medical texts—that it was a combination of therapeutic electric rejuvenation and psychological "mental therapeutics": technological treatment administered by skilled physicians created an expectation for health within patients that somehow became manifest. Beard reportedly stumbled on the idea of mental therapeutics midway through an electrotherapy session when he realized that his battery had died but, rather than stopping, continued the treatment, much to the satisfaction of his patient. Beard was at a lost to explain how the psychological aspect of electrotherapy worked, but it appears to have been similar to what would be known by the mid-twentieth century as the placebo effect.[33]

Although electrotherapy offered temporary relief from neurasthenia, Beard argued, any lasting solution required a fundamental transformation of American society. To begin with, people had to shrug off the expectation that they participate in all aspects of American liberty; this would unburden citizens of anxiety and allow them to excel in fields of their own choosing, an event that Beard believed would lead to an intellectual and artistic rebirth within America. "The very greatest of the world's few great contributions to literature and science, as well as art, have been made not under the patronage of liberty, but under the eyes of kings and beneath the shadow of despotism," he postulated to the readers of the *North American Review*; "Liberty, by tempting the cerebral forces to easy discharge, is the cruelest enemy of ideas."[34]

Neurasthenia's vital role in the future of modern America, Beard predicted in *American Nervousness*, would be to force citizens to reassess and change their society and habits to make a healthier nation. In his view, this was an empowering message as it gave license to those who wanted to dial back ambitious expectations, and freed the mind from needless activity.

Science provided Beard with his organizing principles for neurasthenia, and the public served as his audience and, ultimately, his subject. He described neurasthenia with a narrative that boldly linked anxieties arising from urbanization, technology, politics, the economy, and the workplace (in short, modernization) to create a diagnosis that placed personal health within a sociological context. This was an extremely ambitious program, which he pushed to the point of irritating many colleagues. "If we cannot admit Dr. Beard's claim in its entirety, if we experience repulsion at his tremendous, but unconscious egotism," Roberts Bartholow remarked to his colleagues at the Philadelphia County Medical Society, "we are still compelled to acknowledge that his work [on neurasthenia] is the most important that has appeared. He was peculiarly fitted to differentiate this malady by reason of the quickness and acuteness of his intellect, his power of analysis in its subtlest aspects, and his far-reaching, his omnivorous faculty for related facts."[35] It is not surprising that Beard's medical colleagues gravitated toward his work: his neurasthenia narrative effectively empowered physicians by making them the therapeutic counterweight to an ever-changing modern society. No longer would doctors have to rely on accidents, infectious diseases, and warfare to supply them with patients, because with the neurasthenia diagnosis modern society alone would do the job of generating sickness. From the patient's perspective, neurasthenia indicated a civilized, freedom-loving mind that deserved more leisure.

Despite Beard's belief that the nervousness accompanying modernity helped defend people from other diseases, the neurologist himself fell victim to an infected tooth, contracted pneumonia, and died at age forty-three, while at the height of his career, in January 1883. His wife died a week later, leaving their only daughter an eight-year-old orphan. (The *New York Times* carried a short announcement of Beard's autopsy, an event attended by a handful of physicians curious to learn what caused their colleague to pass away.)[36] Beard's neurasthenia diagnosis was a boon to Americans who suffered from an array of mental and physical ailments but might have otherwise been hesitant to seek help for fear of being stigmatized as delusional or weak. Neurasthenia even carried a degree of distinction, but at the expense of others whom Beard essentially excluded from his diagnosis, including working-class persons, nonwhites, and non-Protestants. Although the single most important influence on how people understood neurasthenia, Beard was by no means the only influence, and the public's and medical profession's conception of the condition continued to develop after he died.

Silas Weir Mitchell (1829–1914)

With Beard's death, another neurologist, S. Weir Mitchell, became the world's foremost medical influence on neurasthenia. Mitchell, whose distinguished career spanned more than half a century, was a consummate physician as well as a successful author, poet, and regional celebrity—a man of status with an elite clientele. Although Beard deserves credit for weaving a compelling narrative around neurasthenia and aggressively promoting the diagnosis, it was Mitchell who affirmed the illness as a distinctly personal, introspective experience that warranted treatments designed to be transformative events of self-improvement. Like Van Deusen, Mitchell recognized neurasthenics as

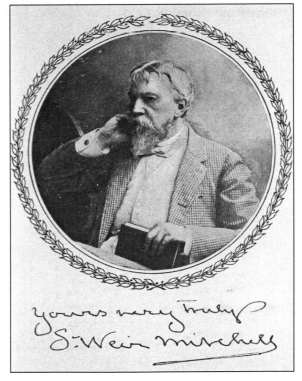

Figure 3 S. Weir Mitchell. Perhaps the most eminent neurologist of his day, Mitchell cultivated an image of himself as a physician-poet who treated the nation's elite for neurasthenia. In the process, he helped make neurasthenia a fashionable illness.

Photo courtesy of the National Library of Medicine, History of Medicine collection.

self-absorbed invalids who made sickness part of their personal identity. He believed that the secret in treating them was to sever their preoccupation with suffering, which he did by refocusing attention away from invalidism and toward other things in life, such as family, art, literature, traveling, recreations, and nature. That Mitchell was a celebrity physician with wealthy clientele is important, as it helped make neurasthenia a distinctive illness in both the public eye and within a maturing medical profession, a profession that Mitchell supported with his lucrative career and influential contacts.

Few people stood at the center of nineteenth-century medicine and culture as completely as did Mitchell. Born a physician's son in 1829, Mitchell followed the family profession and earned his two-year medical degree, specializing in neurology, from Jefferson College in Philadelphia. From there, he traveled to Europe to complete an internship under the renowned French physiologist Claude Bernard, proved himself in America as an able laboratory researcher, and became an expert in nerve damage during the Civil War. Operating out of his hometown of Philadelphia, for over sixty years Mitchell carried on a varied career hardly typical of the narrow specializations that would characterize medicine in the twentieth century. He wrote over 170 scientific papers on topics ranging from reptilian blood pressure to people's fear of cats, as well as four core books on neurasthenia—*Wear and Tear, or Hints for the Overworked* (1871); *Fat and Blood and How to Make Them* (1877); *Lectures on Diseases of the Nervous System, Especially in Women* (1881); and *Doctor and Patient* (1888)—and also penned volumes of popular fiction and poetry. He was a trustee at the University of Pennsylvania for thirty-five years, served as president of numerous professional organizations, and carried on a highly successful private medical practice specializing in nervous women. Although he never held an academic chair of medicine, his writings and active participation in medical societies made him, in the words of the head librarian of the College of Physicians of Philadelphia, "the teacher of those who taught." By the end of the century he had become an elder statesman of medicine, whom *Garrison's History of Neurology* called the "most eminent American neurologist of his time."[37]

Early in his career Mitchell established himself as a dedicated scientist, an ever-important distinction that proved helpful in establishing his medical reputation among his physician colleagues. Unlike Beard, who was largely a social scientist, Mitchell reveled in laboratory chemistry. Operating out of his lab in the basement of his Philadelphia townhouse on the eve of the Civil War, he and partner William Hammond, also a neurologist, made important discoveries concerning the nature of rattlesnake poison that helped produce an antitoxin—just the sort of practical work that made western settlement a little less dangerous and helped to legitimate scientific medicine in the public's eye. Hammond became Surgeon General of the United States at the outbreak of the Civil War and, with Mitchell's encouragement, established Turner's Lane Hospital in Philadelphia, a veterans' hospital dedicated entirely to victims of nerve damage. With his friend Hammond now Surgeon General, Mitchell looked beyond his test tubes to attain a position at Turner's Lane as a contract doctor and a new career as research practitioner. Blocked by alienists from studying patients in asylums, neurologists such as Mitchell took advantage of Turner's Lane and the Civil War's surplus of gunshot wounds, amputations, and distraught soldiers to push the boundaries of neurological knowledge. Results included two landmark publications in neurology written in 1864 by Mitchell with the help of Drs. George R. Morehouse and William W. Keen, *Reflex Paralysis* and *Gunshot Wounds and Other Injuries of Nerves*.[38] Having established his reputation as a first-rate laboratory scientist and a leading neurologist during the Civil War, Mitchell became the natural choice for well-heeled Americans to visit when they felt their peacetime nerves weaken.

While Beard was busy zapping patients with mild doses of electricity, Mitchell stressed the unique aspects of every case of neurasthenia and advocated individually tailored treatment. He advised fellow physicians to learn about the "lives, habits, and symptoms" of each neurasthenic they treated, noting that patients, tortured by the "rack of sickness," made "sad confessions" of things in their lives that weighed them down and drained them of their nervous energy. "The causes of breakdowns and nervous disaster," Mitchell explained in *Doctor and Patient*, "are often to be sought in the remote past." Indeed, in *Doctor and Patient*, written for a popular audience, Mitchell argued that each neurasthenic arrived at his or her condition through a different path, be it the shock of a jilted relationship, the toil of nursing a sick relative, the pressures of education, or the demands of business. "The priest hears the crime or folly of the hour, but to the physician are oftener told the long, sad tales of a whole life, its far-away mistakes, its failures, and its faults," he observed.[39] He reminded people that neurasthenia was not simply the inevitable growing pains of a modernizing society; it was the result of personal experiences within that modernizing society.

Peering into the doctor-patient relationship that Mitchell cultivated is difficult because, outside of general references in his talks and writings, he kept private the personal details of his treatments. Mitchell was an avid letter writer, though, and he corresponded with an impressive array of friends and associates. Some of his friends were also patients, and their letters reveal the personal side of Mitchell's bedside manner. One such woman was Amelia Gere Mason

(1831–1923), a literary critic and intellectual historian from Chicago two years younger than Mitchell. Although Mason was an active, confident, and ambitious woman, neurasthenia sporadically left her lethargic, insecure, and depressed. A particularly devastating bout with the illness in 1882 caused her to "let go and drop the threads of care" and convinced her that her life "had ended." Despondent, Mason traveled to Philadelphia and sought Mitchell's help for the first time. Details of their initial meeting are scant, but one thing is certain: she and Mitchell developed a personal, thirty-year therapeutic relationship that, after Mitchell's death, she told his son was "one of the most valued [friendships] of my life."[40]

According to Mason's letters, Mitchell's strength as a physician derived from his willingness to play the role of confessor, which encouraged patients to speak freely with him. Mitchell possessed an "autocratic" manner while in the presence of patients, and kept an "impersonal" demeanor. Rather than coming off as cold and uncaring, however, his bearing gave off a dispassionate air of authority, one that, Mason acknowledged, made him the perfect partner with whom she could share her thoughts and secrets: "A woman confides to a trusted physician what she could say to no other friend." For someone like her, the doctor-patient relationship and the open communication it entailed provided a source of emotional comfort that helped alleviate the burden of neurasthenia. "What are physicians for?" she asked him. "To serve as a receptacle for human sorrows? Many die, as you know, for the lack of someone to persuade them to live."[41] Mitchell always remained dedicated to medical physiology and believed that good health grew from a strong body, but, as Mason sensed, he also recognized the need for inspiration.

To this end, he advised people who found themselves sinking into a neurasthenic funk to engage in intellectual, creative, and physical activity. Using the example of an unnamed neurasthenic he had known for years, Mitchell argued that her "safeguard from utter wreck" was a "clear and resolute faith" and "a profound and unfailing interest in men and things and books." This, he claimed in *Doctor and Patient*, "gave strange vigor to her whole range of intellectual activities." Mitchell encouraged neurasthenics, especially women, to strengthen and occupy their minds to avoid succumbing to sorrow, pain, and despair. Training the brain to sharpen focus and operate rationally was, in his opinion, one of the best things a person could do to ensure good health. He counseled people to read, write, sketch from nature, paint, learn photography, and keep a diary, as ways to temper their minds and direct attention from depressing topics. Following the bucolic romanticism of Transcendentalists such as Emerson and Thoreau, Mitchell also encouraged neurasthenics to go camping, claiming that the fresh air and fire-roasted food combined with time away from hectic city life would restore mind and body.[42] In short, Mitchell counseled neurasthenics to take control of their lives and improve themselves by developing fortifying interests against self-pity or paralyzing depression.

Therapeutic talk and hobbies might help stave off encroaching neurasthenia, but for those helplessly in the clutches of the disease, Mitchell urged his trademark rest cure. He outlined this cure in the curiously titled *Fat and Blood and How to Make Them* (1877), a thin book written specifically with his medical colleagues in mind. Today, the rest cure is probably best known as the failed treatment that author and economist Charlotte Perkins Gilman underwent for neurasthenia in 1887, a disturbing experience that became the basis of her 1892 short story "The Yellow Wall Paper." In *Fat and Blood,* Mitchell explained how he designed the rest cure for "women of the class well known to every physician—nervous women, who as a rule are thin, and lack blood." Such nervous, upper-class women were indeed the mainstay of Mitchell's clientele during the second half of the nineteenth century, when willowy figures and milky complexions were hallmarks of class and fashion as well as symptoms of a potentially deadly form of neurasthenia that was being diagnosed under the new label *anorexia nervosa.*[43]

Mitchell prescribed the rest cure, it should be stressed, for the most severe cases, for patients in neurasthenic tailspins who were incapable of caring or thinking for themselves. He based this cure on the premise that neurasthenics had bankrupted their supply of nervous energy, were irrational and hysterical, and were beyond the point of being able to benefit from restorative hobbies or activities. In these situations, he believed, physicians needed to create a highly structured environment in which every aspect of the patient's life, including eating, drinking, and movement (bed pans were provided), were regulated for four to six weeks. Feeding was strictly controlled and often began with a week-long milk diet supplemented by coffee, followed by the gradual incorporation of solid foods and hearty soups until the feeding became, in Mitchell's word, "excessive."[44] Social isolation was imperative, as Mitchell believed friends and family would only encourage the neurasthenic's desire for sympathy. Professional nurses were employed to enforce the strict regimen of eating and bed rest, and massages and electrotherapy were administered on a regular basis to keep the muscles toned and lessen the loss of strength.

The rest cure operated on two levels. First, it ensured that neurasthenics ate properly so that they gained weight ("fat and blood") which presumably increased the generation of nervous energy to help pull them from their neurasthenic rut. Second, the rest cure's controlled environment allowed physicians to put patients through a psychological boot camp to strengthen neurasthenic minds weakened by sickness. According to Mitchell, this required "a firm and steady will" ("autocratic," as Amelia Gere Mason saw it) on the part of the physician, so that he could "insure belief in his opinions and obedience to his decrees." Essentially, a physician had to rely on the strength of his force of personality as a tool to subdue, steady, and rebuild the patient's shattered will.

Thus, with a will expertly recrafted by a high-paid medical specialist and a well-fed body nurtured by a strict diet, steady massage, and electrical stimulation, patients who underwent Mitchell's rest cure had every reason to assume that better health lay ahead. To some observers, it was this *assumption* of health that seemed most important, as it was with Beard's electrotherapy. "Hope, expectancy, firm faith that the result must follow the means are powerful adjuvants to massage and electricity," a reviewer of *Fat and Blood* observed. "How the hope long deferred revives again when such a patient is afforded the opportunity to have [Mitchell's] advice and treatment."[45] By placing themselves completely into the hands of the physician, patients who followed through with the rest cure could expect a therapeutic transformation of mind and body that, ideally, would allow them to start life anew, free from neurasthenia. To ensure the best chance for success, Mitchell needed to cultivate what professional medicine for much of the nineteenth century lacked: the necessary authority to garner patients' confidence. It was from confidence in the administrating physician that patients took faith in the medical procedure and expectations of success grew.

One way Mitchell fortified his authority was by leaning on Victorian gender dynamics that granted men authority over women. From his experience, women doctors who in all other ways were perfectly capable practitioners often had trouble securing the necessary obedience from their patients to carry out the regimented cure. He believed that women were naturally more sympathetic and supportive than were men, whom he saw as more rational and decisive. This was a common sentiment during his day, a sentiment that influenced not only the way men and women acted, but also the way people expected men and women to act, thereby making a patient more likely to resist a female doctor who they thought was acting a man's part. Stripped to its barest elements, Mitchell's rest cure relied on gendered role playing to be effective. When Mitchell acted to "insure belief in his opinions and obedience to his decrees," he was not simply playing the role of doctor, but playing the role of *male* doctor to his predominantly *female* patients. Women doctors had troubling emulating this relationship, and similarly Mitchell found it difficult, but not impossible, to reproduce with male neurasthenic patients, whom he deemed considerably more difficult to treat than women.[46]

Mitchell always claimed first and foremost to be a physician, but his public reputation was that of a physician-poet. His literary specialty was stories infused with realistic portrayals of physical and mental infirmities. "I believe that my medical opportunities have been of great value to me as a writer of fiction," he remarked to *Philadelphia Medical Journal* editor George Milbray Gould, "and in every one of my books will be found a picture of some form of disease." All told, Mitchell wrote seventeen novels, including the national best seller *Hugh Wynne, Free Quaker* (1896), in addition to an impressive number of essays, children's stories, short stories, poems, and plays, all of which introduced him to an entirely new audience that might not have encountered him through his medical practice or texts. Rather than detracting from his reputation as a dedicated physician, his literary career contributed to it. "I feel it . . . a great privilege," a fan and patient wrote him in 1902, "to have made the personal acquaintance of one who has such a rare power in the healing art and who at the same time is able to bring entertainment and encouragement to a much wider circle among the reading public."[47]

Mitchell's combination of charm and ability allowed him access to some of the brightest and most successful personalities of his time. "Personally to know S. Weir Mitchell," Dr. William W. Keen remarked, "was a passport in any gathering, not only of medical men, but of laymen." He discussed sculpture with Augustus Saint-Gaudens, theology with Phillips Brook, literature with William Dean Howells, and American history with George Bancroft. He supplied psychologist William James with mescaline, and poet Walt Whitman (a scandalous man by the standards of Philadelphia high society) with a $100 grant, a $15 monthly stipend, and free medical care. He had powerful friends in politics: president-elect William Howard Taft relied on Mitchell's home for lodging and as a place to interview prospective cabinet members, in the days leading up to his inauguration in 1909. Mitchell was friends, also, with captains of industry: steel magnate Andrew Carnegie occasionally dined with Mitchell and at one point asked the doctor what he would do if given $10 million. "I should realize the vain dream of my life—hospital wards and rooms for my Rest Treatment, for the poor," Mitchell replied, playing the role of civic-minded physician. He did not get his money, exactly, but in 1902 Carnegie did appoint him as a founding trustee of his charitable Carnegie Institution (renamed Carnegie Institution for Science in 2007), established with an initial endowment of $10 million. As physician to America's upper crust, Mitchell built, in the words of an early biographer, "one of the most enormous consulting practices in the

United States," which earned upward of $100,000 a year at its height.[48] This was the house neurasthenia built, and it was the envy of American medicine.

Supported by his private practice and familiar with the nation's movers and shakers, Mitchell became a formidable force in shaping the development of the modern medical profession. Beginning in 1856, when he first became a fellow of the College of Physicians of Philadelphia, and ending in 1912, when the Association of American Physicians of Washington made him an honorary member, Mitchell spent fifty-six years adding his influence and administrative capabilities to over fifty national and international organizations, and acting as president to eight of these, including the American Neurological Association, the Association of American Physicians, the College of Physicians of Philadelphia, and the Congress of American Physicians and Surgeons. He also contributed financially, donating thousands of dollars of his personal wealth to organizations and individuals he thought worthy, and became one of medicine's most renowned fundraisers, able to draw then-incredible sums of up to $100,000 from individual donors.[49]

Assuming administrative responsibilities allowed Mitchell to channel money and influence to help the careers of those he thought represented proper scientific medicine. As a founding trustee of the Carnegie Institution, he quickly took advantage of available funds to provide Hideyo Noguchi (1876–1928) and Simon Flexner (1863–1946) with Carnegie Institution grants. Flexner and Mitchell became good friends and Mitchell even invited Flexner to spend his honeymoon at Mitchell's summer home in Bar Harbor, Maine. Both Noguchi and Flexner later became part of the Rockefeller Institute for Medical Research (now Rockefeller University); Noguchi developed a skin test for syphilis, and Flexner became the Rockefeller Institute's first director. (Flexner's brother, Abraham, prepared the Carnegie Foundation's Flexner Report in 1910, arguably the most important document in modern medical education.) As a trustee of the University of Pennsylvania, Mitchell encouraged the career of one of the most esteemed persons in medicine, Dr. William Osler (1849–1919), by spearheading the drive to tempt Osler away from McGill University in Canada and bring him to the United States as the Chair of Clinical Medicine at the University of Pennsylvania from 1885 to 1889. Osler's friendship with Mitchell continued to grow even after Osler left that university to become a founding professor at the influential Johns Hopkins Medical School in 1889, where he established a trend-setting system to educate young doctors: two years of science followed by two years of clinical training. Osler's *Principles and Practice of Medicine* (1892), a book that stressed the scientific nature of medicine, became one of the most influential medical textbooks in the first part of the twentieth century.[50]

Illustrative of Mitchell's use of personal influence to help shape professional medicine is his relationship with Dr. John Shaw Billings. The two knew each other since their Civil War days, and over the years forged an extremely close relationship based on mutual trust, loyalty, and admiration. After the war, Billings stayed in government service as the librarian to the Surgeon General's Office, where he built the foundations of America's modern medical community by compiling the sixteen-volume *Index Catalogue* of medical publications and inaugurating the *Index Medicus*, a monthly guide to current medical literature, which Mitchell helped save from Congressional budget cuts with a Carnegie Institution grant in 1903. In his spare time, Billings designed the plans for John Hopkins Hospital (opened 1889) and edited the *National Medical Dictionary*.[51]

Billings's remarkably productive career left him with little money, a situation Mitchell used his influence to reverse. After failing in an attempt to have Billings made surgeon general under President Grover Cleveland, Mitchell successfully convinced Cleveland to grant Billings early retirement from the army so that Billings could accept a more profitable job as professor of hygiene at the University of Pennsylvania, where Mitchell was a trustee. To help make civilian life more affordable, and in appreciation for his work organizing the nation's medical literature, Mitchell collected a gift of $10,000 from among 254 fellow physicians for Billings and his family. While Billings was still at the University of Pennsylvania, Mitchell worked through his brother-in-law, John Cadwalader, the organizer of the newly founded New York Public Library system, to have Billings made head librarian of the New York Public Library system (with an "unprecedented" salary).[52] Mitchell's friendship and loyalty to Billings illustrates not only the network of influence he had available— Carnegie Institution resources, political pull, university contacts, family sway—but also the type of medicine he supported: a well-informed profession that improved itself by exchanging medical knowledge through journals and by organizing hospitals to work in conjunction with medical schools. It was Mitchell's career in treating neurasthenia—the reputation he acquired, money he made, and influence he gained—that allowed him to shape professional medicine, going into the twentieth century, through promoting colleagues such as Billings.

Mitchell recognized that patients, especially affluent patients, were customers who sought therapy in much the same way they might purchase fashionable literature or clothing. It was the process of meeting with Mitchell, talking with him, having him assess personal problems with a calculating eye and issuing a prescription for self-improvement that was therapeutic. The process was not cheap, and Mitchell had stumbled upon a dynamic that made cost part of the therapeutic process. Edith Wharton certainly recognized this, as her character Pauline Manford demonstrates in *Twilight Sleep* (1937). For Manford, a wealthy middle-aged woman constantly on the lookout for the latest self-improvement therapies, the effectiveness of a treatment is directly proportional to its cost.[53] The more one pays, the higher the expectation for success— and for treatments such as the rest cure, expectations made all the difference.

Along the same lines, the credibility of the medical profession as a whole, and the confidence it inspired in patients, motivated Mitchell, prompting him to contribute resources and influence to building the institutions that shaped the scientifically driven medical profession. The often antagonistic relationship between alienists and neurologists came full circle in 1894 when the American Medico-Psychological Association, the national organization of asylum administrators, asked him to address their convention in the hopes that he could help guide them back into medicine's mainstream. "Asylum life! There is despair in the name as there is in the idea," Mitchell, never one to mince words, declared in a brutally honest assessment of alienists. He urged them to look beyond their asylum walls, engage in "healthy conflicts and honest rivalries" with other physicians, and adopt scientific medicine and experimentation.[54] The neurasthenia diagnosis had enabled him to achieve his position of influence within the American medical community, and so long as he wielded influence, so did that diagnosis.

With neurasthenia, professional physicians such as Beard and Mitchell were able to present the American people with a diagnosis steeped in the sensibilities of the time and that recognized their unhappiness and discomfort while also offering the promise of relief. The diagnosis eliminated some of the stigma of sickness, especially with many of the emotional and mental symptoms associated with the disease, by portraying neurasthenics as casualties of modern society rather than as malingerers or victims of madness. This helps explains why Van Deusen's influence on the development of the diagnosis was limited, his career as an alienist at a public asylum having placed him on the margins of both the medical profession and the type of treatments Americans were looking for during the late nineteenth century.

Beard succeeded in placing neurasthenia into a story of American progress, a narrative that proved attractive to people seeking an explanation for their suffering, while Mitchell developed patient-centered treatments that made being neurasthenic an opportunity to focus on personal issues. Unable to rely on the institutional support of the public asylum system, neurologists like Beard and Mitchell used neurasthenia to cultivate a community of middle- and upper-class patients who could pay for services that strengthened the medical profession. This class aspect of neurasthenia also lent the diagnosis a degree of distinction that encouraged sick Americans to identify with the disease, a phenomenon that turn-of-the-century economist Thorstein Veblen (himself a neurasthenic) would have associated with *pecuniary emulation* and *conspicuous consumption*. After all, neurasthenia's reputation as an illness of distinction could provide those anxious over their social status a de facto place within the respectable ranks of American society.

Beard and Mitchell may have done *too* good a job of making neurasthenia an acceptable, if not fashionable, illness among Americans. By the mid-1880s, the public discussion of neurasthenia had expanded well beyond the control of professional physicians, as marketers and writers began making greater use of the neurasthenia diagnosis in their advertisements and journalistic and literary stories. This caused the meaning of neurasthenia to broaden and become popularized, a process that loosened the conservative connections to class, race, and gender that Beard and Mitchell engineered into the diagnosis (and the treatments). Popularization transformed neurasthenia from a health diagnosis employed by physicians to a phenomenon with boundaries and definitions that were mutually being defined by physician, patient, and popular culture.

Chapter 2

The Popular Diagnosis

The same year that George M. Beard died, 1883, lawyer-turned-illustrator-turned-author Augustus Hoppin released *A Fashionable Sufferer*, a satiric novella about the summer convalescence of a beautiful "Nervous Exhaustionist," an affluent woman in her thirties whose neurasthenic condition, Hoppin noted, was "getting to be rather an envied and enviable lot in life." He explained: "A luxurious civilization has begotten a new order of invalids, who exist on the sweet counsel of their physician and the daily ministration of loving friends." Like Beard and Mitchell, Hoppin attributed the rise of neurasthenia to the modern era, but Hoppin's depiction of the condition, unlike that of the neurologists, was decidedly cynical. He suggested that being a neurasthenic was tantamount to being "rich and fashionable" and implied that those with the condition cared little for social convention. "They are just well enough to go to the opera and the play; just sick enough *not* to go to church."[1] It is not altogether surprising that Hoppin should mix medicine and satire—after all, he had illustrated Dr. Oliver Wendell Holmes Sr.'s *Autocrat of the Breakfast Table* (1858) as well as Mark Twain's *The Gilded Age* (1873)—but to weave a humorous plot around an ostensibly serious illness seems odd, at least at first glance. How had neurasthenia, a medical condition introduced by physicians with great gravitas, become the sought-after malady at the center of a popular satire?

Hoppin's literary use of neurasthenia speaks to the condition's popularization during the period. Beginning with physicians, 250 of whom wrote more than 330 articles on neurasthenia between 1870 and 1910, word about the condition began to spread through late-nineteenth-century America until knowledge of it had become ubiquitous. Although it is impossible today to generate reliable figures as to how many Americans suffered from neurasthenia during the late nineteenth and early twentieth centuries, the condition can nonetheless be considered popularized in that information about, and discussion of, it had spread to the point where neurasthenia had become, according to one turn-of-the-century physician, a "household word."[2] It had become popularized in another sense as well, as medical professionals such as Beard and Mitchell found themselves having to share authority over the parameters of the illness with a wide range of nonphysicians, including advertisers, journalists, and neurasthenics themselves. Pervasive in American society, and beyond the exclusive jurisdiction of professional medicine, neurasthenia was poised, by the 1880s, to go from a medical condition to a full-fledged cultural phenomenon.

Any explanation of neurasthenia's popularization must look at how everyday people, not only physicians, became acquainted with the disease. Aches, pains, fatigue, insomnia, and depression are part of the human condition, but it took a trained mind to identify these experiences as *neurasthenia* rather than something else, such as an imbalance of the humors, a spiritual crisis, or an aspect of temperament. Starting in the 1870s and accelerating into the early 1900s, information on neurasthenia became more widely available to the public, effectively training people to think of their unhappiness and discomfort as part of the neurasthenic condition. Throughout American society, representations and explanations of neurasthenia flourished, ones that blurred diagnostic boundaries normally policed by physicians and, in the process, transformed the disease into a diverse condition sometimes mocked by people such as Hoppin but increasingly recognizable by Americans.

The popularization of neurasthenia took place in four phases, each representing an expansion of the public discussion and knowledge of nervous illness. The years leading up to the 1869 diagnosis of neurasthenia define the initial phase, when European physicians established the parameters of what constituted nervous illnesses and made the links between health and modernity that discussions of neurasthenia would later inherit. The publication of domestic medical and popular health manuals written by physicians about neurasthenia during the 1870s signals the second phase, when neurasthenia first attracted public attention. The incorporation of neurasthenia into the marketing of health care products, generally starting in the 1880s, represents the third phase, when commercial interests blanketed the nation with advertisements and circulars aimed at getting Americans to think of themselves as neurasthenic and thus purchase remedies. The fourth phase, from the 1890s onward, occurred when writers treated neurasthenia as a noteworthy condition and made discussion of the disease part of journalism and literature. With each phase, the reciprocal cycle of shared information about neurasthenia gained momentum, as physicians, patients, and popular culture influenced and were influenced by the others. Ultimately, the popularization of neurasthenia built upon its array of symptoms and lack of a clear pathology, which made the condition protean and responsive to what varied Americans sought in a diagnosis: an opportunity to validate professional services; an advertising tool to sell products; medical flair to spruce up stories; and, ultimately, a way to understand suffering.

Nervousness before Neurasthenia

Despite claims by Beard and others that neurasthenia represented a radically new form of illness that grew out of changes in the lives of civilized people, the diagnosis was actually part of a *tradition* of illnesses linked to the changing ways people lived and worked.[3] In the years before the first articles on neurasthenia appeared, doctors such as George Cheyne (1671–1743), Thomas Trotter (1760–1832), and George Hayden (1798–1857) all connected a perceived spike in nervous diseases to the increasingly urban character of their nations— Cheyne and Trotter were Britons and Hayden, Irish—a theme upon which the neurasthenia diagnosis would later capitalize. They wrote for the literate public, not simply for fellow physicians, and in the process helped shaped both the professional and the popular understanding of what *nervous illness* represented. Newspapers also exposed people to the idea of nervous illness during this period, as stories containing references to such informal predecessors of neurasthenia as nervous exhaustion and nervous prostration eased readers into understanding the role the disease would play in their lives.

Cheyne, a Scots living in England, established the standard description for civilization-induced nervous illness with his 1733 publication, *The English Malady; or, A Treatise of Nervous Diseases*, in which he estimated that a third of affluent patients from his practice near the English resort town of Bath suffered from nervous symptoms such as headaches, anxiety, and depression. The cause for this sudden rise in nervous illness, he claimed, was Britain's economic and cultural success, which resulted in the growth of business-oriented sedentary occupations, late hours, the use of strong liquors, and cosmopolitan diets—providing a "stock of Material for Riot, Luxury, and to provoke Excess." Luxuriated bodies became "soft and yielding," and felt "Pleasure or Pain the most readily." Aggravating the problem was city life, which the doctor deemed too fast-paced, too overcrowded, and too full of debilitating entertainment to preserve health, especially within the enriched capital of London, home to the "most frequent, outrageous, and unnatural" nervous disorders. England's notoriously poor weather served as another supposed factor in nervous illness, as did class, with common laborers (whom Cheyne described as "dull, earthy, clod-pated Clown[s]") having neither the luxury nor the creative acumen to suffer from the English Malady. For treatment, he recommended regimented living involving exercise and a vegetarian diet such as persons of the "middling rank" might eat. Cheyne's book, published in English for the general reading public rather than in Latin for the medical profession, went through six official editions in two years, as well as a pirated Irish edition, and ended up imbuing the concept of nervous illness with traits the neurasthenia diagnosaticians would later adopt, including a distrust of urbanization, a belief in the health benefits of exercise, and the locating of weak nerves in the higher classes.[4]

For over seventy years, Cheyne's *The English Malady* remained the standard text on civilization-induced nervous illness, until Trotter published his *View of the Nervous Temperament* (1807). Trotter reintroduced the subject in stark terms: "At the beginning of the nineteenth century, we do not hesitate to affirm, that nervous disorders have now taken the place of fevers, and may be justly reckoned two thirds of the whole [gamut of illnesses], with which civilized society is afflicted." By doubling Cheyne's estimation of the prevalence of nervous illness, Trotter sought to place *nerves* back on his nation's health agenda. One explanation for this jump in nervous cases, according to Trotter, was that luxury had crossed the class divide and was now enjoyed by Britain's modest classes, rather than by only the "better ranks in life" as in Cheyne's day. By deemphasizing social class, Trotter ended up emphasizing the importance of nationality when it came to nervous health. Britain had become an exceptional nation, he argued, one that "outstripped rival states in her commercial greatness." To some extent, Cheyne had started down this path seventy years before, when he wrote of commercial success and the English malady, but class had loomed too large in his understanding of the condition for nervous illness to be considered wholly nationalistic. *View of the Nervous Temperament* proved mildly successful, going through three British editions and one American edition; one scholar has called it the first book on mental health ever printed in the United States.[5]

With Cheyne and Trotter both blaming modern luxury for the rise of nervous illness, Hayden took the opposite approach by claiming that it was overwork that constituted the prime health threat of modern society.[6] In *An Essay on the Wear and Tear of Human Life* (1846), Hayden insisted that the "unceasing toil, mental labour, and corroding anxiety, while in the pursuit of fame and wealth" in the modern urban environment simply wore people down. Industrialization and British Enclosure Acts during the first half of the nineteenth century led to the rapid growth of the midcentury Dickensian city characterized by impoverished squalor, frenzied effort, and uncertain fortunes, far removed from the easy luxury that concerned Cheyne and Trotter. Business persons were particularly prone to overwork, according to Hayden, as they pushed themselves to dangerous levels—as much out of fear of poverty as from desire for riches, a situation that would only get worse after 1846, when Parliament repealed the Corn Laws and ushered in Britain's era of laissez-faire competitive economics. Looking about his hometown of Dublin, Hayden observed that people tended to "run to extremes. . . . It is the age of locomotion; the demon of the day is ever shouting out, or whispering, 'onward—go a-head!'"[7] Even the phrase at the center of Hayden's book, *wear and tear*, became synonymous with overwork, and a generation later found itself the title of S. Weir Mitchell's popular health manual, *Wear and Tear, or Hints for the Overworked* (1871).

Although health guides written by Cheyne, Trotter, and Hayden provided a pool of public information about nervous illness, Americans in the decades leading up to 1869 encountered *nervous prostration* and *nervous exhaustion* also in the pages of newspapers such as the *New York Times*. Readers learned of John McKay, the Scottish captain of the British vessel *Liverpool*, who killed himself with an overdose of laudanum, an opium-based painkiller, in a fit of nervous melancholia while docked in Brooklyn in 1863. Nervous prostration led to natural deaths as well, as seen in the 1854 obituary of Mrs. Anna Fitzharris of Brooklyn and the 1868 obituary of David Wilmot, Pennsylvanian judge, congressional representative, and author of the Mexican-American War's divisive Wilmot Proviso (1846).

The condition was not always fatal, of course. After the *New York Times* reported that Episcopal Bishop George Washington Doane of New Jersey had taken gravely ill in October 1852, the Bishop's son quickly wrote a clarifying letter to the editor: "He [Bishop Doane] has been suffering from nervous prostration, owing to the fatigue and anxiety of the last two weeks; but having obtained rest, is to-day much better."[8] In 1865, the much-publicized trial of Captain Henry Wirz, the jailor of the infamous Confederate prisoner-of-war camp at Andersonville, Georgia, proved that villains as well as bishops could suffer from nervous prostration. Charged with maliciously subjecting prisoners to "torture and great suffering," Wirz reportedly suffered "increased agony of mind" with each account of "revolting cruelty" the prosecution attributed to him, until he succumbed to nervous prostration, thereby forcing the judge to postpone his trial for four days until Wirz recovered, whereupon he was found guilty and hanged.[9]

As a cause of suicide, natural death, or an inability to appear at trial, nervous prostration and nervous weakness connoted, even in the pre-neurasthenia days, trauma or strain that undermined a person's ability to continue life normally. When Civil War general and postbellum lawyer Thomas Ewing collapsed while arguing a case before the Supreme Court, onlookers attributed the collapse to nervous exhaustion brought on by the gravity of the occasion. The deadly 1864 explosion of a locomotive boiler in Syracuse, New York, delivered a severe head wound to Mrs. Henry Miller, mother of two, and left her with "general" nervous prostration. A story printed in the *Times* even attributed General Meade's reluctance to pursue and complete the destruction of General Lee's army after Gettysburg to the "nervous exhaustion" of his Union troops, a condition the article claimed the Confederates were able to avoid because their dire situation evoked the willpower necessary to fuel their retreat home. But for persons who lived in the slums of New York, home itself was enough to cause sickness, according to an 1859 story. Near the corner of Sheriff and Stanton, the gutters were full of "stagnant, green water," causing the air to be "redolent of decaying vegetables that on a hot day is nauseous to the senses and . . . reek[s] with impalpable and insensible poison." The resulting "[miasma] predisposed all who lived in the vicinity to nervous prostration."[10] These newspaper stories demonstrate that midcentury public knowledge of nervous exhaustion was prevalent enough for writers to use the condition as a reference point when describing job anxiety, catastrophic accidents, the effort of battle, or even the effects of a polluted environment. For those readers who knew little of nervous conditions, the stories built familiarity and contextual understanding.

Although neurasthenia was introduced as a new diagnosis in 1869, the array of symptoms and perceived causes denoted by it had been bouncing around society for years. What united early examples of nervousness were their chronic, sometimes incapacitating, emotional and physical symptoms, such as fatigue, depression, and pain, that made life unpleasant at best and unbearable at worse. Experts such as Cheyne, Trotter, and Hayden generally agreed that nervousness was rooted in the changing way people lived within urban environments, although whether the problem arose from too much luxury or too much work was a debated issue and the source for what would later become contradictions in the popular understanding of neurasthenia. Hoppin's *A Fashionable Sufferer* adopted the luxury explanation of nervous illness, for instance, while Beard and Mitchell where more apt to fault overwork.

Neurasthenia and Popular Health Manuals

After the Civil War, the American medical profession faced two challenges—finding jobs for the glut of decommissioned physicians, and making good on expectations that so-called scientific medicine would yield medical break-throughs. By any standard, the Civil War was a bloody affair. Combat and disease resulted in more than 600,000 Union and Confederate deaths, and more than 14,000 physicians were needed to care for the sick and injured. Although many of these medics returned to their prewar jobs as farmers, clerks, and merchants upon decommission, numerous others sought to build postwar careers in medicine, thereby pressuring the health profession to diversify its services to create additional job opportunities. Neurologists Beard and Mitchell were leaders in this diversification, since they promoted the role of professional physicians as healers of psyches as well as of bodies. The diagnosis of neurasthenia provided the opportunity to combine changes taking place in modern society with common chronic symptoms of unhappiness and discomfort to create a condition that people would look to doctors to treat.[11] But to guarantee a steady stream of patients, physicians needed to convince Americans that their ailments were in fact neurasthenia and did require professional medical care.

Mitchell launched the neurasthenia popularization process with his 1871 book *Wear and Tear*, an unassuming 59-page self-help medical guide written for ordinary Americans that avoided medical jargon and complex explanations, and that relied on the colloquial *nervous prostration* and *nervous exhaustion* to describe the condition, rather than the more technical term *neurasthenia*.[12] Mitchell was clearly ahead of the curve when it came to raising public awareness of neurasthenia, as he published his work just two years after Van Deusen and Beard published their initial articles on the disease and ten years before Beard's *American Nervousness*, the book often credited with securing neurasthenia's place in medical history. In fact, Mitchell dedicated himself to the public discussion of neurasthenia well before engaging his colleagues in a professional conversation over the disease, as his public-friendly *Wear and Tear* came out six years before his more scientific *Fat and Blood*, written expressly for fellow physicians.

Mitchell began *Wear and Tear* in a fashion reminiscent of earlier books on nervousness by asking "Have we lived too fast?" a question answered in the affirmative throughout the volume: "The rate of change in this country in education, in dress, and in diet and habits of daily life surprises even the most watchful American observer," he declared. When it came to faulting the modes of luxury or the modes of work, Mitchell turned his critical eye toward work, as Hayden had done. The process of modernization made Americans "thoughtless sinners against the laws of labor and of rest," according to Mitchell, as they overworked themselves in their drive to get ahead in an urban, capitalistic society beset by the "Dollar Devil." The book was an immediate success, with the first edition selling out in ten days, and a sustained demand over the ensuing fifteen years prompted four additional editions. Not even Mitchell expected his book would do so well. "I am amused to watch the 'Wear and Tear' business," he wrote to his sister Lizzie shortly after the release of the first edition. "No one can be more surprised at this odd little bit of success than I am . . . to have one little flirtation with popular literature written about and talked about from Maine to Georgia."[13] This "flirtation" with popular health literature established what would become a template for the popular understanding of neurasthenia.

Wear and Tear succeeded in combining new developments in medicine with earlier concepts of nervous illness, bucolic romanticism, and healthy common sense. Mitchell placed nervous exhaustion in the grand evolutionary arc of American history through a story of how generations of hardy farmers and pioneers living close to nature had stored up prodigious supplies of nervous energy in their sturdy, robust bodies and vibrant nervous systems. Beginning in the 1850s, this story goes, sons and daughters began leaving farms and the frontier for cities and modern, middle-class lives dedicated to business, education, and professional careers. Fueled by the nervous energy inherited from their parents, this first farm-to-city generation worked long hours, dedicated immense attention to their jobs, and, according to Mitchell, was responsible for the remarkable success of the American economy during the mid-nineteenth century.[14]

Mitchell's narrative held that this economic boom had a downside, as competitive capitalism and intensive education required people to expend inordinate energy to succeed. This was fine for the first generation, which had inherited a large store of energy from its agrarian ancestors. But for later generations of Americans—urban Americans, for whom Mitchell wrote *Wear and Tear*—keeping up with the fast pace of competitive business and education meant overwork, undue wear and tear, and increased risk of nervous prostration. In short, members of the post–Civil War generation of Americans were too ambitious for their own good health. Mitchell believed the climate of the northeastern United States, where the majority of the nation's brain workers lived, was also hostile to good nervous health, its extreme temperatures leaching away nervous energy. He compared the use of vital nervous energy to a bank account: if a person spent more than he or she had saved, then bankruptcy was inevitable. America's urban middle class, according to him, was on the verge of nervous bankruptcy.[15]

A key difference between working in a city and on a farm, *Wear and Tear* pointed out, was that city dwellers relied more heavily on brain labor than physical labor to support themselves. Thinking supposedly used more nervous energy than did physical work, and, to make matters worse, it failed to provide the necessary exercise to keep the body robust and the nervous system toned: "Although it seems so much slighter a thing to think . . . than to hit out with the power of an athlete, it may prove that the expenditure of nerve material is in the former case greater than in the latter." Competitive education, for instance, was thought to be a health threat (especially to adolescent girls) because it forced children to be sedentary rather than physically active and to expend energy on lessons rather than on physical and sexual maturation. Inasmuch as the health of a mother affected the health of her child, this could also harm future generations: "if the mothers of a people are sickly and weak, the sad inheritance falls upon their offspring." Men were also reportedly at risk: they filled the ranks of anxiety-prone businessmen, managers, and clerks faced with putting in feverishly long hours to get ahead. Consequently they risked becoming fixated on work-related problems, developing insomnia characterized by "automatic activity" of the brain, and, unless they took precautions, possibly suffering complete breakdowns and being unable to support their families.[16]

Like many Americans' at the time, Mitchell's understanding of evolution followed the theory of Jean-Baptiste Lamarck, not that of Charles Darwin, meaning he believed species evolved through the inheritance of acquired characteristics rather than through natural selection. For instance, Lamarckians might explain the existence of giraffes' long necks by arguing that the animals had a natural tendency to stretch their necks to get at leaves higher on a tree. As a result of stretching, their necks grew in much the same way an exercised muscle might grow. According to Lamarckian evolution, the offspring of these adult giraffes inherited the propensity to stretch their necks, as well as some of the extra neck length previously acquired by their parents, thereby creating a cycle in which giraffes' necks grew slightly with each generation. Americans such as Mitchell gravitated toward Lamarckism because it offered them the optimistic belief that they could actively manage and influence evolution in a positive way, whereas Darwinism and its stress on natural selection struck them as overly cold and bleak.[17] Mitchell wrote *Wear and Tear* in the hopes of encouraging Americans to take control of their health, and their children's health, by paying closer attention to how they lived, and in the process to help the nation's future evolution.

Other physicians followed Mitchell's lead and produced works on popular health to educate Americans on how to counter the threat of nervous exhaustion and prostration. In 1878, health advocate Dr. Martin Luther Holbrook, proprietor of New York City's Hygienic Hotel and Turkish Bath Institute, published *Hygiene of the Brain and Nerves and the Cure of Nervousness*, a collection of twenty-eight letters, written by notable professionals and public intellectuals, discussing the problem of nervous exhaustion. "In our age nervous exhaustion is in the ascendant," Holbrook declared in his introductory essay. "Our hothouse education promotes it by cultivating the mind at the expense of the body. Our sedentary ways of living promote it. Our haste to get rich, our risks in business, our anxieties, our cares, all help to bring on nervous exhaustion." Transcendentalist Amos Bronson Alcott, poet William Cullen Bryant, *Liberator* editor William Lloyd Garrison, *Godey's Lady's Book* editor Sarah J. Hale, writer and abolitionist Thomas Wentworth Higginson, educational reformer Mary Tyler Peabody Mann, suffragist Elizabeth Oakes Smith, and girls' hygiene author Dr. Mary J. Studley were among the celebrity contributors who acknowledged the threat posed by neurasthenic conditions and who gave personal tips on how to combat nervousness. Readers of Holbrook's work came away with a number of means to avoid errant nerves, including vegetarianism, abstaining from alcohol, daily exercise, limited working hours, developing hobbies, and reading philosophy.[18]

By the late 1880s, physicians had written a sizeable quantity of literature on nervousness for the general public, and, thanks to Beard's 1881 *American Nervousness*, the phrase *neurasthenia* came into general use alongside the older and less formal terms. Mitchell aided in the popularization of neurasthenia by using editions of *Wear and Tear* to publicize his colleagues' works on the topic, including neurologist Horatio C. Wood's *Brain-Work and Overwork* (1882), neurologist Charles K. Mills's "Mental Overwork and Premature Disease among Public and Professional Men" (1885), and Mills's essay "Overwork and Sanitation in Public Schools" (1886). Mitchell's was a very select list of late nineteenth-century titles introducing the issues of nervous weakness and neurasthenia. One could easily have added his own *Doctor and Patient* (1888) (a collection of "lay sermons" written to help women stave off nervousness), California physician H. C. Sawyer's *Nerve Waste* (1888) ("A careful reader can secure useful hints from its pages," a reviewer commented), and Battle Creek Sanitarium superintendent John Harvey Kellogg's *Neurasthenia or Nervous Exhaustion* (1914) ("neither dry nor technical, but couched in terms which anyone may understand," according to an advertisement), in addition to Holbrook's *Hygiene of the Brain and Nerves* and Beard's *American Nervousness*.[19] Thus, encouraged by Mitchell's *Wear and Tear*, physicians during the 1870s and 1880s had published a number of works for popular audiences on the topic of nervous illness, works that coalesced around nervous exhaustion and nervous prostration, conditions subsumed by the neurasthenia diagnosis in 1869 but still useful when communicating with the general public. With *Wear and Tear*, then, Mitchell had brought the old discussion of change and nervous health that had been developed in Europe into post-Civil War America, thereby making it relevant for a population in the process of accelerating its urbanization and industrial and financial economies.

Advertisements, Neurasthenia, and Consumerism

By the 1880s, however, advertisers began to rival physicians as purveyors of popular knowledge of neurasthenia as they incorporated the illness into their promotional literature, especially for health care products. Physicians had already laid the groundwork for neurasthenia-based advertising campaigns during the 1870s with their popular health manuals, which gave neurasthenia and cognate conditions legitimacy in the health care market. Given neurasthenia's array of potential symptoms and its lack of a clear physical cause, it was ideal for the promotion of devices and remedies that promised some form of relief. The narrative explanation for neurasthenia, that is was the byproduct of civilization and modernization, provided a hook for consumers well aware of the changes brought on by invention and big business, while the paradigm of health on which neurologists based neurasthenia—that nervous energy powered the body—proved an easy concept for businesses to co-opt. Using the popular press and mass-produced circulars, marketers flooded America's print media with advertisements designed to spread just enough information about neurasthenia to encourage the public to self-diagnose the condition and invest in remedies.

One of the more curious medical fads that relied on such nervous conditions for sales were galvanized electric belts. Given that neurasthenia was the result of a lack of nervous energy, it stood to reason that recharging the body with energy would eliminate neurasthenia and the lethargy, sexual debility, and pains associated with it. Following Beard's lead in electrotherapeutics, electric belt manufacturers such as American Electrocure Company promised to recharge run-down bodies with a series of galvanized batteries so as to provide "the vim, the strength, the push, the force, the vigor, the power" to drive people through their day and allow them to be as productive and successful as possible. First on Electrocure's list of conditions cured was nervous prostration. Listed for five dollars apiece, Electrocure belts fit snuggly around the waist and contained a series of one-volt batteries that gradually dispensed their charge into the body; customers could also purchase an optional two-dollar "family attachment" providing wires and a conductive band that could be

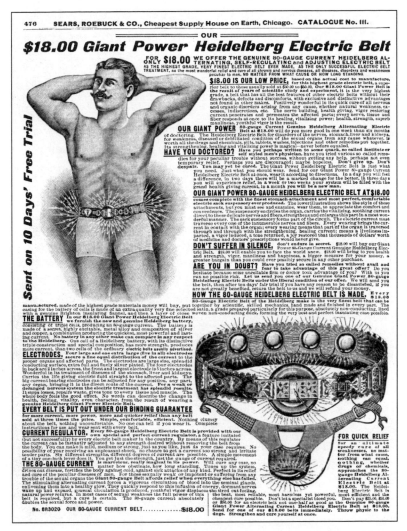

Figure 4 Giant Power Heidelberg Electric Belt advertisement, 1902. Turn-of-the-century entrepreneurs marketed a number of quack medical devices, such as the electric belt, aimed at recharging neurasthenic bodies with vitalizing energy. Advertisements such as this helped spread the word about neurasthenia and worked to make it a popularized condition.

From the *Sears, Roebuck Catalogue* [Chicago: Sears, Roebuck and Co., 1902], 476.

attached to discrete parts of the body that needed recharging. American Electrocure was not alone in the electric belt market and competed with a number of other belt manufacturers, including the German Electric Belt Agency operating out of Brooklyn, with a Suspensory Belt resembling an electrified athletic supporter, and the Heidelberg Electric Belt Company, whose Giant Power Belt boasted an "80-gauge" current for the steep price of eighteen dollars. Advertised by colorful circulars sent through the mail or placed in a wide variety of publications, from Jehovah Witness's *Watch Tower* to the *Sears, Roebuck Catalogue*, therapeutic electric belts were portrayed as the perfect health accessory to help modern Americans combat neurasthenia, their modern national disease.[20]

The fad of electric belts was almost insignificant in comparison with the most profitable part of the late nineteenth-century commercial medical market, proprietary medicines. Often referred to as patent medicines, proprietary medicines were big business, and neurasthenics represented a potentially lucrative body of customers. Census figures show that in 1859, on the eve of the Civil War, the nation's patent medicine manufacturers earned $3,500,000, a number that would increase twenty-fold to $74,500,000 by 1904. A turn-of-the-century observer estimated that patent medicines were so economically successful that their total value exceeded the combined worth of the nation's production of chocolate, flavoring extracts, axle grease, beet sugar, glue, castor oil, lard, kindling wood, cosmetics, and gun finishing. This late-century surge in these medicines grew through a confluence of events, including the proliferation of newspapers, an increase in national education and literacy, manufacturer-friendly patent laws, reduced postage costs, and a general rejection by Americans of the excessive bleeding and purging associated with nineteenth-century professional physicians and their heroic medicine. The Civil War itself was also critical to the development of the patent medicine market, as people eager for the latest news developed daily reading habits that exposed them to the barrage of advertisements and circulars on which medicine manufactures relied to sell their products.[21] Equally if not more important were the hundreds of thousands of people who suffered from emotional and physical injuries sustained in a conflict that tore apart bodies, families, and personal lives. Postwar America urgently needed its nerves soothed, and the nation's pharmaceutical industry was eager to oblige.

Unlike physicians, who worked out of offices and hospitals, patent medicine manufacturers had to rely on marketing materials to establish their presence within communities. A marketing expert from the 1880s estimated that it took $50,000 in advertising to create a demand for any particular medicine, let alone to produce, bottle, and ship the product, and failure to invest in advertising would sink an otherwise profitable medicine company within five to six years. As an 1898 exposé on patent medicines observed, the old reasons for taking medicine—to relieve fevers and malaria—were quickly disappearing as backwoods areas thought to cause illness were developed. "Advanced civilization," the article noted, brought with it new ailments including those of a "vast army of up-to-date neurasthenia victims" willing to consume medicine in "surprisingly great quantities." Advertisements aimed at exploiting this market lined the pages of newspapers and periodicals across the nation; the 1897 *Sears, Roebuck Catalogue*, for example, dedicated twenty pages to list more than four hundred medicines claiming to cure the gamut of human and animal ills.[22] Buying pharmaceuticals had become as normal as ordering clothes or hardware, and, as their use spread, so did word about neurasthenia.

Given their need to advertise, ambitious medicine manufacturers resembled publishing firms more than they did traditional pharmaceutical companies. The Doctor Miles Medical Company, for instance, owned its own press and bindery, employed more typesetters than chemists, and in 1889 distributed over 100,000 16-page booklets aimed at selling their bottled neurasthenia cure called Nervine. To help ensure their ads were not simply thrown out or used as kindling, drug companies often wove their advertisements into promotional almanacs that contained calendars, space for shopping lists, indexes of useful home remedies, and even handy strings for conveniently hanging the almanacs from a nail. In St. Louis alone, half a dozen pharmaceutical firms produced over twenty million almanacs annually. Medicine manufacturers cast a wide net by reaching out to immigrant groups and publishing in multiple languages. The Hostetter Company had nine different editions of its almanac, each for a different ethnic group, while Dr. D. Jayne and Sons marketed its "Family Medicines" almanac in twelve languages—German, Welsh, French, Spanish, Swedish, Norwegian, Portuguese, Bohemian, Dutch, Italian, Chinese, and, of course, English. All told, from the 1870s through the 1890s the number of almanacs published yearly by the patent medicine industry provided at least one almanac for every two Americans, and spread rudimentary information about diseases and industry products throughout America's immigrant groups. When Ayer's almanac proudly claimed to be "second only to the Bible in circulation," it very well may have been right.[23]

Creating name recognition was only one goal of advertisers; the other was to garner health care dollars by educating Americans about illnesses such as neurasthenia so that they had the confidence to self-diagnose and medicate themselves. The United States Medicine Company's booklet "Dr. Dunlop's Family Practice: A Hand Book of over 100 Common Diseases Giving Symptoms and Treatment" was typical of this informative approach. The handbook provided page after page of ailments, each with its own description and prescription. It cleverly characterized chronic nervousness as "annoying from the fact that nervous persons really suffer much more than they get credit for," thus establishing the idealized Dr. Dunlop as a sensitive, sympathetic caregiver. The handbook listed fretfulness, fear of impending evil, hot and cold flashes, and faintness as symptoms of nervous exhaustion, which the United States Medicine Company claimed sufferers could counter with sea baths, cold showers, milk punch, and the daily use of its trademarked Cascara Compound.[24]

This strategy of presenting a pithy breakdown of symptoms, causes, and treatment became standard in patent medicine circulars. In the 1892 "Warner's Safe Cure Almanac," Warner and Company blamed poor blood for neurasthenia and recommended daily use of their Safe Cure and Safe Nervine to ward off symptoms. The Shaker Medical Company's 1887 *Almanack* linked nervous prostration with indigestion and prescribed Shaker Extract of Roots, which they claimed increased bile and restored tone to the stomach, liver, and kidneys. To help drive home the pharmaceutical message of self-diagnosis and self-treatment, the *Sears, Roebuck Catalogue* ran a banner at the bottom of the page in its drug section, reminding consumers to "Save Exorbitant Doctor Bills" by treating themselves with medicine.[25] A little knowledge goes a long way in advertising, and the more familiar people became with recognizing symptoms associated with neurasthenia, the more likely they were to self-diagnose and to self-prescribe a bottled medication.

When it came to developing a marketing campaign around products to recharge neurasthenic bodies, few companies succeeded like Doctor Miles Medical Company of Elkhart, Indiana. Established in 1884, Miles Medical produced a line of "restorative" medicines that included Restorative Tonic, Restorative Blood Purifier, Heart Restorative, and its best seller, Restorative Nervine ("a brain and nerve food and medicine, which soothes and quiets the brain and nervous system while it furnishes nourishment and strength").[26] In a free 1891 publication, "New and Startling Facts for Those Afflicted with Nervous Diseases," the Miles Company claimed to have sparked a "new era in medical science" that would "revolutionize the theory and practice of medicine as effectually as the steamboat and railroad have the old modes of travel, or as the telephone and telegraph have the past methods of communication." Miles's simple "grand truth" was that "Nerve-Force is to medical science what Electricity is to the mechanical world." Following the logic outlined by Beard in his theory of nervous energy, the company proclaimed that each organ in the human body "is but a part of an electrical machine" that needed to be energized to remain healthy. To drive this point home, company publications provided an illustration, "Modern Medical Science: Neuropathy," that depicted a man whose transparent body revealed organs superimposed by images of various machines: the brain was a series of batteries; the eyes were electric lights; the

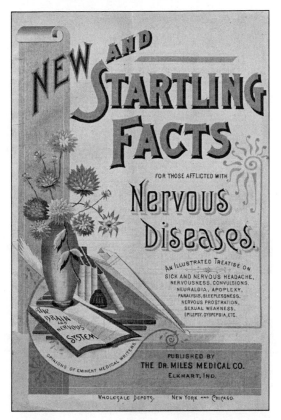

Figure 5 Dr. Miles Medical Association (1891). Pharmaceutical companies published booklets like this as a way of getting people to self-diagnosis with neurasthenia as the first step towards self-medicating with proprietary medicines.

Advertising Ephemera Collection—Database #A0433; Emergence of Advertising On-Line Project; John W. Hartman Center for Sales, Advertising & Marketing History; Duke University Rare Book, Manuscript, and Special Collections Library; http://library.duke.edu/digitalcollections/eaa/.

lungs were electric fans; the feet were trolley cars, and so on.[27] Just as these electrical devices would malfunction if lacking in power, so people's bodily organs would malfunction, according to Miles Medical. The cure was Nervine, convenient bottles of therapeutic energy delivered directly to a patient's door without the help, or added expense, of a doctor.

The effectiveness of patent medicines at treating neurasthenia should not be completely discounted. Physicians tended to advocate electrotherapy, rest cures, and lifestyle changes designed to recharge the body's nervous energy or remove neurasthenia-inducing anxiety; medicines often contained drugs that combated the symptoms of the illness. Since manufacturers at the time

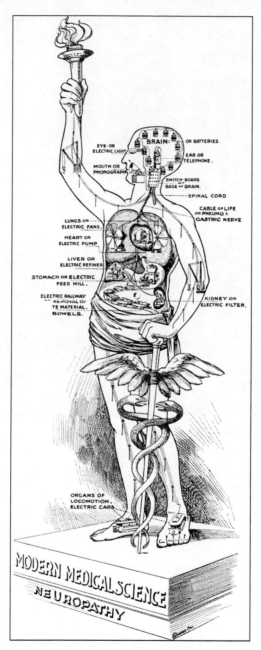

Figure 6   Dr. Miles Medical Association (ca. 1894). As a way of coaching Americans how to think of themselves as broken-down neurasthenics, pharmaceutical companies such as Miles' Medical circulated images, such as this, that recast the body as a collection of electric-powered machines.

Image courtesy of Advertising Ephemera Collection—Database #A0412; Emergence of Advertising On-Line Project; John W. Hartman Center for Sales, Advertising & Marketing History; Duke University Rare Book, Manuscript, and Special Collections Library; http://library.duke.edu/digitalcollections/eaa/.

considered the ingredients of their products trade secrets, the exact composition of these medicines is not entirely clear. Only after 1906, with the passage of the Pure Food and Drug Act and the subsequent establishment of the Food and Drug Administration, were manufacturers required to print ingredients on product labels. Scholars today agree, however, that the active ingredients of patent medicines tended to be sedatives, stimulants, and psychotropic drugs, some of the most common being alcohol, bromides, caffeine, cocaine, marijuana, and opium. Many compounds also contained iron, known at the time to combat the exhausting effects of anemia, and vegetable concentrates that we now know to be rich in vitamins, although the role of vitamins in nutrition was not fully understood until the first part of the twentieth century.[28] Given some of the ingredients, addiction was always a potential danger with patent medicines and may help account for their impressive sales. Yet because they were packaged as "medicine," these products allowed America's Victorian-era upstanding citizenry to self-medicate while keeping a public semblance of sobriety.

The information about nervousness and neurasthenia found in patent medicine circulars often paralleled what professional physicians at the time were saying about the condition. Circulars stressed how neurasthenia was a product of modern civilization, overwork, competition, anxiety, and the "secret vice" of masturbation. "What Kills Americans!" the title of an article in the 1887 Shaker medicine almanac proclaimed, before listing the guilty causes: "Fast Living—Reckless Eating—Hard Drinking—Poor Sleeping—Social Jealousy—Political Ambition—Violent Passions—The Race for Money."[29] Such piggybacking on what physicians had already written about neurasthenia worked to reinforce the parameters of the condition in people's minds, thereby making it a more familiar and intuitive illness, something worthy of self-treatment via a proprietary medicine.

Eager to cultivate as large of a market as possible, medicine advertisers generally aimed for the rich, poor, and middle classes simultaneously. For instance, the 1887 *Almanack* published by the Shaker Medical Company not only contained plentiful medicine advertisements but also featured two informative exposés. The first, "The Peaceful Life of the Shakers," painted an idyllic picture of the modest religious group, describing them as the "most successful communists in the world." The second article, "The Young Money-Makers of America," contrastingly provided illustrated biographies of famous, even notorious, capitalists such as railroad magnate Cornelius Vanderbilt, financier Jay Gould, wealthy statesman William Waldorf Astor, and meatpacking titan Philip Armour. Whether you aspired to the communist piety of Shakers or the capitalist riches of robber barons, the *Almanack* wanted your attention and your business. Also stressing the uniform effectiveness of their products, the Miles Medical Company was comfortable placing a testimonial from a "prominent business man" from Pennsylvania alongside testimonials of an Arkansas pastor, a Spanish dancer, and an Ohio veteran.[30] Identifying subtleties and variations within neurasthenia cases were not that important for pharmaceutical advertisers, as they did not want to risk muddling the thrust of their message: You might be neurasthenic, so buy our product.

Neurasthenics, though, were infamous for being indecisive and often needed the reassuring guidance of a medical expert to guide them back to health. Addressing this problem, Miles Medical and other pharmaceutical companies established "treatment by mail" programs whereby sick people could mail in descriptions of their ailments and expect a response from a physician. Until the practice was outlawed in 1922, company experts supposedly reviewed each letter and issued a prescription "according to the latest scientific researches in medical science": "Nowhere else," a Miles circular claimed, "do ailing people receive the same skillful treatment, the same careful consideration, or the same prompt attention for so reasonable a charge." Even while Miles Medical stressed its rational, scientific approach to treating neurasthenia, other companies, most notably Lydia Pinkham (a very profitable patent medicine producer), gave the impression of offering compassionate, homespun health advice through the mail. This proved to be particularly effective at attracting female customers who believed that the male-dominated medical profession was ill suited to cure women's nervous conditions brought on by menstrual cramps, pregnancy, and menopause.[31] Thus, by the turn of the century the American pharmaceutical industry had established a marketing system that catered both to neurasthenics who had faith in scientific medicine and to those who distrusted a medical profession dominated by northeastern-educated male physicians.

Treatment by mail programs also functioned as a market research tool that allowed medicine companies to keep tabs on health demographics so as to more effectively advertise and cultivate a demand for their neurasthenia products. Company circulars sometimes provided standardized forms designed to elicit information. For instance, the Toledo, Ohio, manufacturers of the Parker Remedy for Men urged individuals to complete a questionnaire with their name, address, age, weight, occupation, marital status, and whether or not they suffered from any of a long list of symptoms, including loss of "vitality, strength and vigor," "nervous and weak" feelings, melancholia, sleeplessness, painful or difficult urination, constipation, indigestion, or piles (hemorrhoids). Inquiries were also made into personal habits such as the "secret vice" of masturbation, or tobacco or alcohol use.[32] Questionnaires provided insight into the health and personal lives of Americans, allowing companies such as Parker Remedy to hone their advertising to incorporate the various symptoms of unhappiness and discomfort that Americans at the time were experiencing. This created a dynamic cycle of information that allowed sick people to affect the way medicine marketers understood neurasthenia, which in turn produced advertising that influenced the way the larger population of neurasthenics understood their illness.

Letters from customers (sometimes heavily embellished or written outright by ad writers) also provided fodder for punchy testimonials that gave a personal touch to the way patent medicine manufacturers spread information about neurasthenia. Most testimonials were short, often providing only an individual's name or initials, the person's hometown, and a brief statement about the effectiveness of the medicine being advertised, although some circulars showcased lengthier testimonials. Claiming to present "Honest Words from Honest People," Miles Medical Company distributed a mock newspaper complete with illustrations and dozens of stories, mostly dated 1892, of those cured by the company's Restorative medicines. For instance, Mrs. Viola Mamanis of Milton, Iowa, claimed that "overwork and grief" had brought her to the "verge of insanity": "The world was dark to me, my life was a burden, and at times the desire to end my existence entered my mind." Her case confused doctors, she stated, because, although her physical health was "apparently good," her mental condition was "deplorable beyond expression." Solace came from five bottles of Miles's neurasthenia treatment, Restorative Nervine, which, she said, made her "as happy as a lark."[33] Testimonials in the same publication also noted that Nervine cured the weight loss of businessman J. C. Stephen, the headaches of Col. C. W. Dean, the crippling spasms of the Spanish dancer Cyrene, the epilepsy of a Missouri girl, the prostration of an overworked Ohio housewife, and the heart problems of a Cornelia Graumlich of South Bend, Indiana. By connecting such a disparate array of people and symptoms to a single cure for nervous exhaustion, patent medicine testimonials helped to open the floodgates for the popularization of neurasthenia. Nearly any ailment could be a sign of the illness, it seemed, and nearly anyone could suffer from it.

As illness had a way of motivating people to spend money on products, marketers found during the late nineteenth century that neurasthenics constituted a profitable clientele. Not only did advertisements for health products such as electric belts and proprietary medicine put *neurasthenia* and related terms in the public view, but circulars also listed symptoms and coached people on how to think of themselves as neurasthenic. Medical products were just the tip of the iceberg, as advertisements in newspapers, magazines, and circulars peddling all sorts of late-century products and services began cashing in on the neurasthenia trade. By the turn of the century, references to neurasthenia were appearing in promotions for health resorts, bicycles, railroads, dried breakfast cereals, "invigorator" corsets, exercise weights, and self-help books. Neurasthenia had become a ubiquitous and commercialized condition. Yet, though marketers increased neurasthenia's profile as a medical condition and helped provide a name for people's suffering, they remained part of a somewhat rough-hewn commercial culture that at the turn of the century was still a generation away from achieving the level of cultural influence advertisers would enjoy from the 1920s onward. Even so, by the 1890s, neurasthenia had made the jump from selling products on the side of the page to being at the center of attention in American newspapers and magazines.

Neurasthenia as Topic of Interest

While physicians wrote domestic health manuals on neurasthenia and advertisers used the condition to help sell their products, by the 1890s writers were making neurasthenia the subject of news and popular literature. This was not an entirely new development, as newspapers like the *New York Times* had been incorporating conditions such as nervous exhaustion and nervous prostration into stories even before the 1869 development of a neurasthenia diagnosis. As the turn of the century neared, the number of such stories increased, as did neurasthenia's role within them. Writers helped make this diagnosis part of common knowledge, a topic of news and human interest familiar to millions who might otherwise have paid little attention to popular health manuals or remedy advertisements.

At the end of the century, mention of nervous illnesses continued to appear in obituaries, especially in explaining suicides. For some neurasthenics, death proved the desired alternative to institutionalization. Max Meyer, an Alabama dry goods merchant of "extremely delicate health" who for years suffered from insomnia and neurasthenia, jumped to his death from a window early in the morning in 1894 upon hearing that his brothers intended to place him in an asylum. Frances Titsworth, the neurasthenic wife of a cashier, similarly killed herself by jumping from the sixth story of a private sanitarium. "While the nurse who was attending the sick woman yesterday morning had her back turned," the *New York Times* reported, "Mrs. Titsworth got out of bed, threw up the window, and leaped to the ground." Even absent the looming presence of institutionalization, newspaper obituaries made it appear as though neurasthenics had a proclivity for defenestration. Such was the case of

Ralph S. Lansing, a thirty-year-old Treasury Department lawyer who "deliber-
ately walk[ed] toward the window, opened it, and before anyone could inter-
fere stood for an instant on the sill and sprang into space" from the ninth floor
of his workplace. "His nervous system and mind were not what they should
be," Lansing's physician commented to reporters, "and I am not surprised at
what has happened." Readers of the *Times* would have noticed that neurasthenia's deadly influence touched a wide range of victims and could cause Harris
Rosenberg, a downtown pawn broker, to jump in front of a subway train as easily as it could drive Charles Whitney, a respected Wall Street broker, to put a
bullet in his head.[34]

Attributing suicide to neurasthenia had a way of reducing the stigma of the
act, as the real culprit became the disease and the deceased became a victim.
Cornelius Jeremiah Vanderbilt, whom the *New York Times* described as the
"discarded" son of shipping and railroad magnate "Commodore" Vanderbilt,
shot himself in the head in 1882 while convalescing in New York's Glenham
Hotel. "It was nervous prostration," Judge Edwin O. Perrin, a family friend, told
the *Times*. "Spells of that nature came upon Mr. Vanderbilt very frequently and
he was utterly irresponsible at those times." Vanderbilt's personal physician,
Dr. George Terry, agreed: "No troubles could have prompted him to kill himself, and it must have been due entirely to the state of his health." Readers of
the *Times* learned that the betrayal of a spouse could also cause the development of neurasthenia and subsequent suicide, as in the case of Mrs. Wallace
Widdicombe, a performer who, under the stage name Muriel Nelson, had established herself as an accomplished composer, violin player, and actress. After
testifying in court during divorce proceedings as to her husband's infidelities,
she returned home "weeping bitterly" and, in the early morning, killed herself
with a bullet to the right temple. "When her domestic unhappiness came upon
her," the newspaper explained, "her nerves went to pieces and she became
a victim of neurasthenia." When Albert Pulitzer, of the Pulitzer newspaper
conglomerate, fatally shot himself in front of a mirror while in Vienna in
1902, reports claimed that the suicide was "unexpected even to his private
secretary"; according to Pulitzer's physician, Dr. Pollack, the newspaperman
"became the victim of neurasthenia twenty years ago through overwork. . . .
Lately his malady developed into a persecution mania, a sudden attack of
which may have prompted the suicide."[35] By invoking neurasthenia as the
cause of suicide, and then attributing the neurasthenia to something readers
could sympathize with, such as rejection by a loved one or overdedication to
work, these accounts discouraged readers from fixing the blame on the people
who killed themselves.

Neurasthenia also became a way for newspapers to explain other sorts of bizarre, destructive behavior. When Mrs. J. R. Waters, the fifty-year-old wife of a successful insurance underwriter, murdered her twenty-two-year-old daughter Agatha with a pistol in 1906 and then turned the gun on herself, the front-page story attributed the violent actions to a "temporary fit of insanity" brought on by neurasthenia. Another murder-suicide captured the attention of Americans in 1909, when wealthy New Jersey landowner David Henderson gunned down his daughter, Martha, and then shot himself, while at a family party at a fashionable Parisian restaurant. Rumors that Henderson was furious with his daughter for having an affair with an Italian were denied by the family, who focused attention instead on Henderson's despondency and his subtle references to suicide made during the last year of his life. "A clear case of neurasthenia," the *New York Times* reported to readers looking for an explanation for such a violent crime committed by an East Coast notable.[36]

Despite being known as the "American disease," neurasthenia's ability to generate erratic and self-destructive behavior was not limited to the United States. A 1909 *Times* story about the Czarina of Russian reported that this empress's neurasthenia sometimes produced "absence of mind," which prevented her from recognizing friends or servants. Another reported side effect of her neurasthenia was that she was "haunted . . . by an indescribable fear"—a prescient premonition for a woman who would be executed with her family by Bolsheviks eight years later. American readers learned that the Czarina was not the only Russian who suffered from neurasthenia. An overseas correspondent for the *Times* reported that "neurasthenia is claiming an ever-increasing number of victims in all sections of St. Petersburg society." Aristocratic Russian neurasthenics had a penchant for elaborate suicides and homicides, such as hosting champagne parties wherein one bottle was laced with a lethal dose of opium. Or, if more action was desired, two neurasthenics armed with pistols would enter a darkened room where they traded shots with each other. Between the poisoned bottles and blind gunfights, Slavic neurasthenics gravitated—within the pages of the *New York Times*—toward variations of the Russian roulette theme.[37]

In many cases at the turn of the century, neurasthenics did not have to die or kill to make the news; the breakdowns of famous people became news in themselves. New York playboy Lloyd Aspinwall's neurasthenic collapse made the news in 1893, with the reporter taking the opportunity to gossip about Aspinwall's clothes, age, and spendthrift ways. When Helen Keller, the deaf and blind disability activist, had a neurasthenic breakdown and could not attend her 1904 Radcliffe graduation, the *New York Times* reported it on the front page. The *Times's* competitor, the *New York Daily Tribune*, carried a multi-installment feature on Charles Schwab's 1902 debilitating neurasthenia, reportedly brought on by his overexertion as president of U. S. Steel Corporation, the largest company in the world at the time. "Physicians fear serious recurrence if the steel trust president does not take a rest," the *Tribune* warned, covering Schwab's life from his initial breakdown, through his recuperative European trip aboard his yacht, to rumors of his forced retirement. The feature made for a lively story that provided readers with pictures from inside Schwab's handsome Atlantic City mansion, an itinerary of his trip to Europe, and an explanation of how the demands of running the world's largest business had outpaced the ability of one of America's most able tycoons.[38]

By this period, too, neurasthenia had become a topic of progressive journalism, covered by mainstream, general-interest magazines. Emblematic is the *North American Review*'s 1892 article "Do We Live Too Fast?" by Dr. Cyrus Edson, the chief inspector of the New York Board of Heath. The essay, with its title evoking the question asked by Mitchell twenty-one years earlier in the introduction to his popular health manual *Wear and Tear*, warned readers of the dangers posed by modern society. Edson claimed that, over the previous generation, America's free-market economic system had forced people to ratchet up the pace of life to a "fearful speed": "The American works harder than does any other man or woman on earth. His business is always with him, he has no rest, no cessation, no relief from the strain." Even leisure was strenuous, as Americans demanded "the most exciting" books, "sensational" dramas, intense sports, yachts that "fly over the surface of the sea," and nearly anything "all intense, all startling, all sensational." Edson contended that this active American life wore on the nerves of women more than on those of men, because women usually exercised less, suffered the strain of childbirth, and generally had more highly wrought nervous systems. Edson also suggested that it was "impossible to overrate" the detrimental effect on people's nerves of the "periodical press" as it reported on every anxiety-inducing business failure, famine, and "alarming trend"—an ironic observation for an article on the alarming trend of neurasthenia. Concern over the nation's constant supply of unnerving news clearly shows Beard's influence on Edson, who also echoed Beard's belief that neurasthenia represented the tragic result of American greatness. The "very elements in ourselves that have made us great, the push, the drive, the industry, the mental keenness, the ability and the willingness to labor," Edson explained, "contain in them the seeds of national death."[39]

Thinking it "impossible" to eliminate the enervating aspects of modern life, Edson and the *North American Review* argued that all Americans must strengthen their ability to withstand modern strain: "We must, as a people . . . , understand this: that while we drive the brain we must build the body." This process of health-building needed to begin early in life and include plenty of fresh air and physical education. "We must teach our children to exercise until it becomes a habit," Edson told Americans, "and we must choose a form of exercise which is adapted to persons of middle age." Making exercise a life-time, family-oriented event was foremost in Edson's mind: outdoor sports should be "judiciously" encouraged by parents, and dumbbells, chest weights, and other exercise equipment should become "part of the furniture" of every household. Girls, in particular, needed fresh air and exercise to help them grow into young women with "bright eyes, clear complexions, stately carriages," and the strength to bear healthy children. Modern America would not lose the race between nations, Edson insisted, so long as citizens followed the mantra: "Build up the body, build up the body!"[40]

The *North American Review* was one of numerous magazines that catered to turn-of-the-century middle-class sensibilities and increasingly turned a critical eye toward social problems. It is hardly surprising that editors sought stories about neurasthenia, the quintessential modern disease merging work, rest, and health into a single social issue. In 1893 *McClure's Magazine*, the journal that would become a bulwark of muckraking journalism, featured an interview with Mitchell (mistakenly introduced as "Samuel" rather than "Silas") in an article by Edward Wakefield, "Nervousness: The National Disease of America." There were indeed many neurasthenia-based articles: *The Eclectic Magazine of Foreign Literature, Science and Art* taught a lesson on "Nerves and Nervousness" (1894); *The Century Magazine* addressed the question "Are Nervous Diseases Increasing?" (1896); *Scribner's Magazine* looked inside the home with "Domesticated Nervousness" (1898); and *Outlook* incorporated children into the equation with "Nervousness and Fatigue in the School Room" (1899).[41] Although these articles may not fit squarely into the category of muckraker journalism, they nonetheless were part of the progressive movement that sought to identify and alleviate social problems through research, publicity, and reform. In so doing, the pieces deepened the reading public's knowledge of neurasthenia.

The topic of neurasthenia went beyond journalism to become embedded in American literature. Books such as William Marrs's *Confession of a Neurasthenic* (1908) and Margaret Cleaves's *Autobiography of a Neurasthene* (1910) provided readers a personal look at the despondency, the fear of being misunderstood, and the obsessions that could plague neurasthenics. On the other hand, Hoppin's *A Fashionable Sufferer* (1883) and O. Henry's *Adventures in Neurasthenia: Let Me Feel Your Pulse* (1910) provided readers with a more comedic portrayal of neurasthenia as an illness of choice more suitable for satire than sympathy. Short stories addressed neurasthenia from many angles, with Charlotte Perkins Gilman's chilling "The Yellow Wall-Paper" (1892) illustrating how treatment for neurasthenia under Mitchell's rest cure was akin to being locked in an asylum and could be more traumatic than the illness itself. Theodore Dreiser's "Scared Back to Nature" (1903) provided a light-hearted remembrance of the author's recovery at a health camp populated by a colorful collection of neurasthenics led by a stern taskmaster. The anonymously written "Autobiography of a Neurasthenic" (1910) gave a soul-searching account of how overcoming neurasthenia meant redemption as a husband and father. Neurasthenic characters littered turn-of-the-century fiction, including Mitchell's own manipulative Octopia Darnell in *Roland Blake* (1886), Frank Norris's pensive Presley in *The Octopus* (1901), and Edith Wharton's fallen socialite Lily Bart in *The House of Mirth* (1905).[42] Literature contextualized neurasthenia within people's lives and created model neurasthenics, archetypes that readers could emulate, ridicule, or use as a touchstone.

By the 1890s, neurasthenia had become a multifaceted fixture in American journalism and literature, one that people could not ignore. The illness connoted drama, as news stories conjoined it with suicide and violence; the considerable number of notables associated with the condition also bestowed a certain level of distinction. People learned of the many symptoms, causes, and treatments of neurasthenia from the pages of popular magazines that saw it as a topic suitable for features. All this print dealing with neurasthenia had the effect of reducing the medical profession's authority over it and popularizing the condition so that everyday people felt comfortable identifying with it.

Self-Identifying with a Popularized Neurasthenia

Within a generation of Beard's first article on neurasthenia and Mitchell's popular *Wear and Tear*, public knowledge of the disease was expanding under its own momentum as a deluge of reported symptoms, causes, and cures flooded American society. Physicians were quick to notice. In 1894, Dr. I. N. Love of St. Louis published an essay in the *Journal of the American Medical Association* lamenting neurasthenia's prominent place in the imaginations of sick Americans. In particular, patients startled Love by their tendency to approach physicians with the *intention* of being diagnosed with neurasthenia, and he commented that "to a certain degree it has become the fad on the part of the American public to elect to be placed under" that label. Yes, Love admitted, these patients may have been victims of weariness, but weariness was not the same as the medical diagnosis of neurasthenia. A decade after Love's diatribe, neurologist Charles L. Dana published an article in the *Boston Medical and Surgical Journal* recognizing that the condition had become a cliché, and even gave a tongue-in-cheek example of European physicians who routinely diagnosed neurasthenia as soon as an American patient was announced. This story was only partially a joke: it also reflected the belief that neurasthenia had become a perfunctory diagnosis, one readily understood and accepted, if not outright expected, by patients.[43]

As information about neurasthenia expanded, so did the types of patients who self-identified with the condition. In addition to influencing the clients of private physicians such as Love and Dana, popularization also influenced patients who relied on free clinics, such as the dispensary run by Cooper Medical College in San Francisco.[44] In 1895, one F. Finck visited the Cooper clinic complaining of weakness, exhaustion, back pains, lack of ambition, and headaches brought on by worrying and personal troubles. According to the attending physician, Finck had been "reading up on his case" and found "all of his symptoms recorded in the books." The diagnosis: neurasthenia. A forty-year-old Russian fruit seller suffered from seminal emissions, constipation, and general numbness, all made worse, according to clinic staff, by anxiety experienced after he read "a great deal about his troubles." The diagnosis: neurasthenia. Similarly, a brooding forty-eight-year-old blacksmith from Iowa worried that he was acting "unnaturally," a condition the clinic partially blamed on the "great deal of quack literature" that the man read. The diagnosis: neurasthenia.[45] To a point, popularly available information on neurasthenia acted as a self-fulfilling prophecy: the more people learned of the condition, the more likely they were to become fixated on the disease and emulate its symptoms. Although such patients most likely did not waltz into the Cooper Clinic to the extent the more affluent caricatures drawn by Love and Dana visited private physicians, they nonetheless demonstrate that people could be influenced by the widely available literature on neurasthenia.

Popularization did not solely mean that patients were familiar with their condition; with time, physicians also became comfortable locating neurasthenia in populations apart from the middle- and upper-class white Protestants to whom Beard had initially tethered the illness. In the 1870s Mitchell had been surprised to find neurasthenic laborers while dispensing free medical care out of the Philadelphia Infirmary for Nervous Diseases. A generation later, researcher Sidney Schwab identified neurasthenia as the most common neurological diagnosis among Jewish garment workers in St. Louis, afflicting from 25 to 30 percent of seven thousand neurological patients studied over a ten-year period. Eventually physicians also began identifying neurasthenia among black patients. In a speech before the National Medical Association (the national organization for black physicians; the American Medical Association enforced racial segregation), Dr. J. A. Robinson admitted that, for years, doctors like himself had followed Beard's lead and only diagnosed neurasthenia in patients of a "highly intelligent nature" but had eventually realized that neurasthenia affected American society as a whole, white and black, brain-worker and laborer. The root of the problem, he claimed, was the city and its promise of easy wealth and leisurely living, which lured people away from modest yet healthy farm work. Similarly, Irving Rosse, a well-traveled neurologist, found neurasthenia afflicting blacks in increasing numbers after the Civil War, as the abolition of slavery and migration to cities such as Washington, D.C., led them to more modern lifestyles. Far from the influence of the city, Rosse reported, he even found evidence of neurasthenia among the Eskimo, while on expedition to the Bering Strait; this observation threatened to severe the link between neurasthenia and urban modernity altogether.[46]

Everyone was a potential authority on neurasthenia, because no one was an absolute authority on the disease. Physicians such as Mitchell began the popularization process with popular health manuals written for common folks in the hopes of getting Americans to identify everyday problems with nervous exhaustion deserving of medical attention. Quickly adopting the neurasthenia diagnosis as a marketing tool, advertisers sought to guide people toward finding relief in purchasable medical remedies. By the turn of the century, newspapers and magazines became yet another source of neurasthenia knowledge as they used the illness to add depth to stories, explain otherwise inexplicable behavior, report on the latest celebrity breakdown, and be at the center of feature stories. Americans suffering from chronic pain, depression, insomnia, indigestion, impotence, infertility, headaches, or anxiety faced a motley assortment of health advice that agreed on little other than that these symptoms were part of a relatively modern condition known as neurasthenia.

The popularization of neurasthenia also had a way of empowering people to *personalize* the condition. Neurasthenia's symptoms—the unhappiness and discomfort—prompted people to reflect upon their lives for clues that might reveal a source for their suffering, a source more profound than the clichéd explanations of luxury or overwork.

Chapter 3

The Search for Inspiration

Neurasthenia and Therapeutic Spirituality

During an evening sermon a few days after Christmas 1907, Episcopal bishop Samuel Fallows made an announcement of interest to the neurasthenics in his Chicago congregation: "I have arrived at the conclusion that mentality, when based upon a trust in religion, is a powerful aid toward the cure of all functional nervous disorders." Hypochondria, sleeplessness, indigestion, melancholia, hysteria, drug habits, irritability, anger, fear, indecision, and neurasthenia could be conquered, Fallows claimed, by tapping into the "triumphant power of the mind." This power, according to the bishop, relied on "Christian psychology" that harnessed "mental and spiritual forces" of which the "dominant note is religious and scientific faith." "This is not a new or sudden fancy of mine," he said, with a reportedly whimsical smile. Indeed, Fallows was an established lecturer of physiological psychology at Bennett Medical College and had been working with colleagues in Boston in the hope of linking "all churches irrespective of creed in this beneficent effort" to heal victims of nervous disease. It was an important endeavor, Fallows stated, and nothing less than the "imperative demand of the age."[1]

In claiming that "religious and scientific faith" could help cure neurasthenia, Bishop Fallows identified himself as part of a wide-ranging therapeutic religious movement whose advocates sought to combine soul searching with psychology to create health, happiness, and comfort. The melancholy emptiness that often accompanied neurasthenia had a way of prompting people to introspectively reexamine their lives in search of reasons for their affliction.[2] Despite claims by physicians and pharmaceutical companies that the condition was rooted in the physical world and nervous energy, many neurasthenics found their suffering too emotionally wrenching to be purely physical and looked to alternative explanations. For them, neurasthenic ennui pointed to a debilitating spiritual malaise that grew out of a maladjusted mind, with cure to be brought about through reflection, meditation, and self-help.

Therapeutic spirituality was a diverse movement, inspired by the mid-nineteenth-century teachings of mesmerist Phineas P. Quimby, and which found its way into people's lives through numerous books on the topic. Generally known as New Thought, this movement was basically decentralized and defined by a genre of literature, though it did have organizational manifestations such as the Church of Christ, Scientist, and the early twentieth-century Emmanuel movement, of which Bishop Fallows was a member. Practitioners of therapeutic spirituality did not always see eye-to-eye on issues of health, spirituality, and scientific medicine—in fact, they were often in open disagreement with one another—but what united them as part of a single movement was the belief that mental and bodily health were inextricably linked to faith. Therapeutic spirituality proved remarkably effective at treating the unhappiness and discomfort of neurasthenics, but in so doing it attracted the ire of many within the medical profession, who objected to what they thought was the encroachment of religion into the domain of physicians.

By the turn of the twentieth century, a professional turf war of sorts broke out as a dedicated group of doctors waged a legal, professional, and public relations campaign against practitioners of therapeutic spirituality. In response, proponents of therapeutic spirituality, such as leaders of the Emmanuel movement, sought to legitimate their methods by attributing their spiritual strategies to leading figures within the scientific medical community, such as S. Weir Mitchell. Despite this very public conflict between organized medicine and spiritual healing, a number of physicians, including James Jackson Putnam, learned from their neurasthenic patients the effectiveness of a personal religious philosophy. The case of Susan Elizabeth Blow, a patient of Putnam's, illustrates the profound influence that a patient could have on her physician's understanding of disease and therapy, and provides insight as to how neurasthenics could heal themselves through spiritual self-help. Faced with the dilemma of wanting to protect the integrity of professional medicine yet incorporate the effective components of therapeutic spirituality, Putnam and others worked to reconcile the conflict by establishing *psychotherapy* as a middle ground.[3]

The New Thought Movement

Neurasthenics might have been well known for lethargic languishing, but their minds were often abuzz with wild thoughts in search of order, and assaulted by waves of despair from unclear sources. Although some neurasthenics sought to ignore their troubled minds through intoxicating patent medicines or highly structured rest cures, others dedicated themselves to regaining control over their minds to minimize mental anguish and support themselves with positive thoughts. After all, it stood to reason that if despairing thoughts made neurasthenia unbearable, then reassuring thoughts might help alleviate it. During the late nineteenth century a therapeutic movement developed that explored the possibility of restless minds healing themselves through nothing more than reflective thought. Popularly known as "mind cure," the movement referred to itself as New Thought and drew heavily upon the nation's neurasthenic population looking for relief and an explanation for their suffering.

The therapeutic roots of New Thought trace back to the movement's founder and inspirational guide, Phineas P. Quimby (1802–1866). While working as an apprentice clockmaker, Quimby fell ill with consumption and nearly died from heroic doses of calomel (a medicinal mercury compound) administered by physicians. Following the suggestion of a friend, in 1833 he took a carriage ride outside town in the open air and, upon returning, came to the sudden realization that he was cured. Reflecting on his newfound health, he concluded that sickness came from *thinking* he was sick, while health came from thinking he was healthy. The implications of Quimby's experience were profound, as they meant that both health and sickness originated in the mind rather than the body. Frequenting physicians contributed to illness, he posited, because the professionals focused on what it meant to be sick rather than on what it meant to be healthy.[4]

An encounter with an itinerant mesmerist, a few years later, introduced Quimby to the theory of animal magnetism, the supposed ability of some persons to influence others through the use of hypnotic power. Quimby then combined the concept of animal magnetism with his theory of health to found a doctoring ministry that would cure the body by treating the mind. Quimby described his therapeutic strategy: "My practice is unlike all medical practice. I give no medicine, and make no outward applications. I tell the patient his troubles, and what he thinks is his disease, and my explanation is the cure. If I succeed in correcting his errors, I change the fluids of the system and establish *the truth or health. The truth is the cure.*"[5] By vocally describing their ailments, Quimby developed a sympathetic connection with his patients that was vital to convincing them that their illness was merely a state of mind, and that changes in the mind could prompt changes in the body. Making health synonymous with truth was important in that it gave his treatment the weight of a moral imperative. The teachings of Christ, Quimby contended, contained God's truth and the secrets of healthy thought; consequently, just as Christ could cure through sympathetic interaction with the sick, so too could Quimby and others who studied the supposed science behind Christ's wisdom. During the nineteenth century, a time when the concept of science was in flux, Quimby's approach could be considered scientific inasmuch as it relied on careful analysis of Biblical texts combined with the collection of anecdotal evidence.

Quimby died in 1866, but his followers wrote a series of books that carried therapeutic spirituality to the neurasthenia-prone generations that followed, books that became the basis of New Thought. Warren Felt Evans, a Swedenborg minister whom Quimby helped cure of a neurasthenia-like nervous affliction, become an early leader of the movement and penned a number of texts on mind cure, including *The Mental Cure* (1869), *Mental Medicine* (1872), and *Soul and Body* (1876). Julius Dresser and his wife, Annetta Gertrude Dresser, elaborated on Quimby's therapeutic philosophies in *True History of Mental Science* (1887) and *The Philosophy of P. P. Quimby* (1895), two books that combined with the work of Evans to give shape to the New Thought community. New Thought writers typically combined Quimby's teachings with Emersonian Transcendentalism to develop a new religious therapy unaffiliated with any established congregation (a scholar of the movement called it a "religion of the printed word") and dedicated to bringing inspirational relief to American neurasthenics.[6]

With New Thought, neurasthenics found a spiritual explanation for their suffering and instructions on how to use mental power to shed reliance on physicians and medicines. Although the people and ideas behind New Thought date back to before the 1870s, its name arose in the 1890s to replace the generic label that the movement previously went by, "Christian Science," after Mary Baker Eddy, founder of the Church of Christ, Scientist, copyrighted the phrase. Martin A. Larson, a follower and historian of New Thought, described the movement as "a revolt against the old and conventional dogmas of the historic religion of the Western World." He compared the impulse behind New Thought with Swedenborgianism and the Shakers, two religious sects originating in eighteenth-century Europe that attracted followers in mid-nineteenth-century America by melding optimistic utopianism, mysticism, and Christian teachings. By the turn of the twentieth century, New Thought had more than one million followers and over one hundred monthly and weekly periodicals.[7]

Horatio Dresser (1866–1954), son of Julius and Annetta, was a leading figure within New Thought and helped bring the movement into the American mainstream by developing a universal theory of religion, health, and philosophy for self-help. In 1907, at age forty-one, he earned his Ph.D. at Harvard, working with William James and Josiah Royce, two of the world's leading authorities on pragmatism. Dresser impressed James, who described Dresser's ideas as a "systematic philosophy of life" that ought to be appreciated for its "concrete therapeutics." Dresser's first mind-cure book, *The Power of Silence* (1895), began as a series of Boston lectures and became a resounding success that went through fifteen editions in eight years. "There is a new demand made upon man," Dresser observed in his introduction, "to understand himself in the light of all the causes that have operated to produce him, his thought, his daily experience, his joy and suffering." According to the author, people were not individuals alone and adrift in the universe but rather were part of a larger spiritual collection shepherded by God. The key to good health and happiness was listening to one's soul, one's true nature, because it was a conduit through which God's power flowed: "Wherein man is adjusted to it, he is already free from suffering. He moves with it, and knows how to be helped by it."[8] The difficult part of life, according to Dresser, was understanding one's soul amid the daily distractions one encountered. Education, fashion, religious dogma, personal expectations, and the expectations of others all worked to misdirect one away from one's soul and toward arbitrary, unhealthy standards. Hence, the "power of silence" in the title of his book referred to the vital process of tuning out society's harmful static so one could hear the soul's energizing message.

Illnesses such as neurasthenia had a purpose, according to Dresser, because their agonizing symptoms served to prod people into aligning their lives with the soul-based life God intended them to live. Dresser contended that, if people would only live according to their natures and listen to their souls, there would be no poor health. Yet sickness existed, and, reflecting the progressive sentiment of his time, Dresser reasoned that, just as the suffering of the poor and the grief of crime victims prompted societies to enact more enlightened policies to ameliorate poverty and reduce crime, so too should people's emotional suffering stand as motivation to help guide them toward a more perfect understanding of their souls and the universe. "Suffering, then, is intended to make man think. The final meaning of suffering is hope . . . the message of the Spirit as it speaks to us in moments of despair, in times of trouble, throughout life, throughout history, in all evolution, is a grand inspiring Hope."[9] His was an inspirational message designed to pull neurasthenics back from the precipice of despair and instill a necessary optimism.

The linchpin to Dresser's spiritual philosophy was belief in an Immanent God who served as a wellspring of unlimited therapeutic power. Dresser equated his Immanent God with Ralph Waldo Emerson's "Over-Soul" and stressed how the process of tapping into this power was highly individualized and required personal introspection rather than formulaic beliefs or the charismatic influence of another. "I advocate that interpretation of life which places the responsibility largely on ourselves," Dresser explained, "which teaches us not to lean on systems of thought and on people in whom we believe and whom we permit to do our thinking for us, but encourages us to look within and to find in our own souls an ever-present resource." The cure for poor health, he posited, was for people to help themselves, in Emersonian fashion, by reclaiming control over their thoughts and beliefs, shrugging off external influences, and becoming more self-reliant.

In the end, it was incumbent upon individuals to adapt to the rest of society, rather than the reverse. "Can we not become adjusted to the situation as it actually is, and stop this continual rebellion, this sense of disease and lack of harmony with the inevitable?" Dresser asked. "Possibly our suffering is largely unnecessary, and is caused by our own attitude." Although it may seem that Dresser is unfairly blaming neurasthenics for being ill, his message also discouraged passivity and sought to empower people to take control of their lives. The message offered health and power via the mind and spirit, an attractive prospect for those who otherwise felt weak or victimized by neurasthenia. Dresser even titled the last chapter of *The Power of Silence* "Self-Help," a hallmark phrase of the New Thought movement and a reaffirmation that people's spiritual connection to God empowered them to make personal improvements.[10]

Therapeutic Religion—Christian Science

For the most part, spiritual therapeutic movements such as New Thought were decentralized, relying more on loose principles than on strict doctrines, and encouraging open participation. There was, however, a sizable institutional dimension to turn-of-the-century therapeutic religion, which coalesced around the treatment of chronic illnesses such as neurasthenia. From the Quimby tradition came Mary Baker Eddy (1821–1910) and the Church of Christ, Scientist, a therapeutic congregation that worked to define Christian Science as a distinct organizational doctrine apart from the more loosely defined New Thought movement. Like many in this tradition, Eddy was critical of professional medicine and championed her Christian Science church as an alternative. Physicians countered with accusations of charlatanism and claims that Eddy endangered the lives of those in her congregation. Tensions came to a head by the turn of the twentieth century and American neurasthenics found themselves caught in the middle.

Eddy had founded the Christian Scientists' Association in 1876 (it became the Church of Christ, Scientist in 1879) as an organized religion built on the premise that health was ultimately a spiritual matter. Eddy had initially been a follower and champion of Quimby, who had helped cure her of her own neurasthenia-like illness. Shortly after his death, Eddy hurt herself in a fall and, while recovering, had a religious epiphany in which she believed she had discovered the secrets to Christian Science. Within ten years, she had enough followers to found her church, and thereafter she developed a Christian Science orthodoxy, policing its boundaries by distancing her teachings from those of Quimby's and by excommunicating followers who challenged her authority or associated too closely with the rest of the New Thought movement. From Eddy's initial congregation of 26 in 1879, the church grew to 86,000 members by 1906 and to 202,000 by 1926.[11]

Under Eddy, Christian Science became American's premier therapeutic religion, one that claimed to cure any ailment, from cancer to broken bones. "The same power which heals sin heals also sickness," Eddy declared. She believed that people were in essence pure thought—spirits—that created their own reality, including their bodies, their successes, and their failures. Christian Scientists looked to the Bible and Eddy's personal revelations for direction on how to realize the potential of the mind so as to repair their bodies, improve their lives, and reconstruct their realities. "You say that accidents, injuries, and disease kill man, but this is not true," Eddy explained. "The life of man is Mind. The material body manifests only what mortal mind believes, whether it be a broken bone, disease, or sin."[12] In practice, Eddy sought to recast the world from a physical place to a spiritual place.

Eddy built Christian Science as a health care alternative to professional physicians, whom she claimed perpetuated illness by filling unsuspecting people's minds with negative thoughts of disease and sickness. She outlined her therapeutic spiritual beliefs in *Science and Health* (originally published in 1875), which served as the doctrinal handbook of Christian Science and contained numerous accounts of persons cured by Eddy's methods. Like Quimby before her, Eddy thought poor health arose from a misguided mind, and good health could be achieved by following proper thoughts, as revealed through the teachings of Jesus Christ. In 1881, she established the Massachusetts Metaphysical College to teach people the art of Christian Science healing with a program of six to ten lessons. At $300 the tuition was steep, but those who completed the course were certified as Christian Science practitioners and could begin careers as healers and congregational leaders, earning in some cases well over $5,000 a year. For those who could not afford a certified

Christian Science healer, Eddy's *Science and Health* reportedly contained enough therapeutic wisdom to provide relief. "Some years ago I was pronounced by a professor of *material medica* . . . a neurasthenic," a testimonial in the 1906 edition of Eddy's book read. "I was almost constantly taking medicine and had in all eleven physicians who undoubtedly did their best, but without avail, notwithstanding almost all known drugs . . . [and] very many patent medicines." Whereas doctors and medicine failed, the author of this testimonial, C. E. M. of Philadelphia, found a cure for his neurasthenia in *Science and Health*, claiming simply that the "book has done the work and I am a well man."[13]

Even though men such as C. E. M. found relief through Christian Science, it was among American women that Eddy's church gained most of its supporters. At the beginning of the twentieth century, women comprised over 70 percent of Christian Science membership, a greater proportion than the national average of just under 60 percent for all church denominations. One reason for this high rate of female membership undoubtedly came from Eddy herself, who encouraged women to assume leadership roles within the church, a position at odds with that of most American denominations, which relied on male leadership. Also, Eddy's religious language was often deferential to women—for instance, her use of the phrase "Mother-Father" in reference to God, and her tendency to valorize womanly qualities while associating men with sinfulness. In addition, Christian Science was considerably more egalitarian when it came to health care. Although the number of women enrolling in medical school and earning MDs was increasing during the late nineteenth century, men still dominated the mainstream medical profession, and women found it very difficult to earn medical educations and build careers. Christian Science, however, encouraged the enrollment of women in its health classes, so that by 1890 women comprised 75 percent of all Christian Science practitioners, a number that would grow to 89 percent by the time of Eddy's death in 1910.[14] Finally, for neurasthenic women who otherwise liked to keep busy, active, and sober, Christian Science's focus on therapeutic spirituality must have represented an attractive alternative to undergoing six bed-ridden weeks of Mitchell's rest cure or to risking intoxication and addiction by consuming alcohol- and drug-laden medications.

As Christian Science grew in popularity, so did its body of critics. Eddy came under fire for being obsessed with money and her church a money-generating cult that garnered more than $4 million for her personal use. In his 1910 book *Faith and Health*, Charles R. Brown, dean of the Divinity School at Yale University, dedicated a chapter to "The Loss and Profit of Christian Science," wherein he claimed the church's healing colleges churned out quack certificates—reportedly, class attendance was not even required—simply to collect the $300 tuition. Stories of Christian Science healers allegedly conning money out of sick and dying patients made headlines in turn-of-the-century American newspapers. For instance, the *New York Times* provided extensive coverage of the 1901 court case involving the will of a Helen C. Brush, deceased, who left the bulk of her estate of $90,000 to the First Church of Christ, Scientist. Relatives of Brush accused the church's pastor, Augusta A. Stetson, of using healing sessions to manipulate Brush into making the church her prime beneficiary.[15] The court eventually ruled in favor of the church, but the case nonetheless brought acerbic accusations and negative publicity to Christian Science.

In other cases, grieving family members accused Christian Science healers of malfeasance that resulted in wrongful deaths. Such was the case of the wife of Santiago Porcella, who died of consumption while under the care of a Christian Science healer and whose husband accused the church of misleading the family into thinking the condition was improving when in fact it was becoming terminal. "It was murder," he told reporters. Tuberculosis was notoriously difficult to cure until reliable antibiotic treatments developed in the 1940s, and professional physicians were often no better at curing the disease than were Christian Science healers, but what particularly irked medical doctors was the bold claim that Christian Science could cure *any* condition. During a discussion in front of the Quid Nunc women's club of New York, Dr. John B. Huber challenged Christian Scientists to provide evidence that they had successfully treated "typhoid fever or malaria or pneumonia, and cases believed by physicians to be incurable," and concluded that the religious movement constituted a "psychopathic epidemic" of charlatans convinced of their own god-like powers. Huber's fellow discussant, professor of law and medicine W. A. Purrington, was more direct in his assessment of Eddy's form of religious healing, calling it "vain, greedy, ignorant, vulgar, and profane."[16]

Although practitioners of scientific medicine generally scoffed at Christian Science's ability to cure physical illnesses such as tuberculosis, by the turn of the century increasing numbers within the medical profession recognized that Christian Science had in fact stumbled upon an effective way of curing neurasthenia. Neurologist Charles L. Dana of Cornell Medical College thought that the sect's therapeutic potential came from encouraging sober, balanced living. Some nervous sufferers "get a tremendous amount of help," he wrote in a 1900 *New York Times* feature, "from that small amount of religion in Christian Science which lends itself to self-control and not to foolishness." In a speech before the Boston Society for Medical Improvement five years earlier (1895), Harvard neurologist James Jackson Putnam identified a powerful mental therapeutic within Christian Science that he argued was akin to the psychological power of suggestion. Drawing on the ideas of the transcendentalist Emerson and the pragmatists Josiah Royce and William James, Putnam argued that the mind and body were closely connected and that neurasthenia symptoms usually originated from morbid, depressing thoughts: "It is essential to form powerful associations in the mind, which have a strong sense of hopefulness and cheerfulness as one of their elements." Christian Science did this, Putnam argued, by using "verbal suggestion" to implant the "seeds of hopefulness and confidence" into patients' unconscious minds and thereby redirect neurasthenia-inducing morbid thought toward positive, health-inducing thought.[17]

With his 1895 speech, Putnam called on his fellow practitioners to take seriously and explore the therapeutic potential of psychological suggestion, upon which he argued New Thought and Christian Science relied. Physicians such as Mitchell had already gone down this path, Putnam pointed out, with the rest cure, which Putnam claimed was effective not because of the gaining of fat and blood (as Mitchell had initially argued), but because it was an arduous process that ended with a powerful declaration of health by the physician, a ritual of sorts that inspired patients into believing they were well. Putnam argued that the medical profession needed to go further to win back the confidence of neurasthenic patients who were defecting to become "disciple[s] of the Christian Science or Mind Cure": "In a sense I grudge the irregulars every case that they win from us, be they few or many, because I believe that with a deeper knowledge of human nature, a better understanding of psychology, a wider range of methods and greater skill in applying them, we could cure more of these patients ourselves."[18] There was nothing inherent in religion that healed people, according to Putnam; there was no rejuvenating spiritual energy. Rather, it was psychology, specifically the therapeutic power of suggestion, that provided the force to treat neurasthenia. Reflecting the pragmatism of his Harvard colleagues, Putnam insisted that American physicians needed to put aside their prejudice against Christian Science and look past their educations in biology and physiology to accept that otherwise "quack" treatments such as hypnotism and religious mind cures might, for neurasthenia, actually offer effective therapies.

Combining Medicine and Faith—the Emmanuel Movement

Tensions between professional physicians and advocates of religious therapies came to a head when the Emmanuel movement began a campaign to treat neurasthenia in 1906. The Emmanuel movement started at Boston's venerable Emmanuel Episcopalian Church in 1905 as a way of bringing together the medical knowledge of professional physicians and the philanthropy of religion to treat tuberculosis among the urban poor. Led by Reverends Elwood Worcester (1862–1940) and Samuel McComb (1864–1938), the anti-tuberculosis campaign featured regular checkups administered by physicians and a series of rooftop camps that allowed tuberculosis victims and their families the opportunity to live in fresher air above the city's tenements and streets. Widely considered a success, the tuberculosis campaign led to the decision by Worcester and McComb in 1906 to embark on a similar program to treat nervous disorders. Nearly half of their patients suffered from neurasthenia, but many also suffered from alcoholism and from other nervous complaints. Patients who wished to participate underwent a rigorous selection process; for instance, from September 1908 to January 1909 approximately five thousand people applied for help, but only one hundred were chosen for treatment.[19]

The Emmanuel movement sought to make health care part of the responsibility of the modern church. Neurasthenia proved the ideal condition to target because medical studies such as Putnam's had demonstrated that neurasthenia responded well to moral therapy and the therapeutic use of suggestion. Worcester and McComb were no amateurs when it came to mental therapies. Worcester held degrees from Columbia and the General Theological Seminary in New York, as well as a Ph.D. in philosophy from Leipzig, Germany, where he worked with Wilhelm Wundt and Gustav Fechner, two pioneers in the field of experimental psychology. McComb, who was Irish, earned his Ph.D. in psychology at Oxford and interned under neurologist and early psychotherapy advocate Sir William Graham. Worcester and McComb secured the early support of some of medicine's finest names, including Isador Coriat (follower of Sigmund Freud, and pioneer in group therapy), Richard Clarke Cabot (Harvard Professor of Clinical Medicine and Social Ethics), and Putnam. The program involved weekly public lectures on issues of mental and physical health, medical examinations by physicians, and clergy-led counseling sessions designed to help patients regain confidence and take steps to improve their lives. Christian teachings stood at the core of the program, as they were seen as providing a template for wholesome, responsible living that would help ground neurasthenics and infuse their lives with meaning.[20]

Although Emmanuel organizers were eager to distance themselves from Christian Science, whose advocates they considered too radical in their claim that health was entirely a mental perception, the Emmanuel movement can nonetheless be grouped with Christian Science and New Thought as a reaction to nineteenth-century scientific medicine rooted in the material world. "We believe in the power of the mind over the body," Worcester announced in the introduction of the movement's 1908 handbook, *Medicine and Religion*. He explained that the United States was experiencing a great spiritual awakening characterized by a renewed belief in prayer and the "confident expectation that religious and spiritual states can affect health." A seismic cultural transformation was afoot, he wrote, from which Americans would emerge aware of the limits of rational, scientific thought and increasingly recognizant of the benefits offered by faith. "If the nineteenth century was materialist and critical," Worcester posited, "the first half of the twentieth century promises to be mystical and spiritual." It was time for the "physician and clergyman" to combine their forces for the "benefit of the community."[21]

Worcester and McComb bid for the public support of America's reform-minded progressives by writing articles in popular magazines and traveling the nation to teach classes on the movement's therapeutic strategy. For nearly two years, starting in 1907, *Good Housekeeping* served as the movement's informal mouthpiece. Editors proudly announced that their magazine had "been chosen by Rev. Drs. Worcester and McComb as the periodical through which the good news shall be spread, accordingly it will assist clergymen, physicians and others in establishing centers and introducing the work in their churches or districts." The *Good Housekeeping* articles often contained testimony of people helped by the movement, such as Miss B., whom Worcester aided in becoming a "bright, clever, and entertaining woman," and Mr. Packard, whom McComb helped to overcome his "utter hopelessness and despair." Within a year, stories on the movement ran in many other journals, including *Century, North American Review, Current Literature, Popular Science Monthly, Outlook, American Magazine, Independent, Review of Reviews,* and *Ladies' Home Journal.* Worcester and McComb also led an intensive, three-week workshop in 1908 to teach 140 other clergy the methods of religious healing, in the hopes that they would take the knowledge back to their congregations. By the fall of that year, the movement had spread to Chicago, Brooklyn, New York, and San Francisco.[22]

When it came to the origins of the Emmanuel movement's therapeutic strategy, Worcester stressed that the blueprint originated from none other than the sage of neurasthenia treatment, Dr. S. Weir Mitchell. Years before Worcester founded the movement in Boston, he had served as rector of St. Stephen's church in Philadelphia and there had struck up a friendship with Mitchell. The elder neurologist and the young cleric shared interests in psychology and health, and they discussed the importance of religion as a regulator of the human psyche. "I would like to tell you that I regard our friendship and our conversations in Philadelphia as choice blessings in my life," Worcester later

wrote to Mitchell. He called Mitchell his greatest mentor, telling the neurologist, "There is no one in the world whose advice I should value as highly as
yours." In a 1909 letter to Mitchell, composed while on a train to California to
help spread the movement to the West Coast, Worcester gave the Philadelphia
neurologist ultimate credit for the Emmanuel movement's neurasthenia
campaign, telling him that it was all the "direct result of your influence and
example and your writings and conversation." Worcester had said much the
same thing to the press, and was quoted giving Mitchell credit for the idea
that "religion and therapeutics ought to go hand in hand, and that such a combination would be invincible."[23] Mitchell's name still carried weight in 1909,
and, if Worcester could have grafted the Emmanuel movement to Mitchell's
reputation, then the movement would have had de facto credibility.

Looking back on Worcester's deferential letters to Mitchell, it is likely that
the rector was also trying to curry favor with the neurologist amid the medical
profession's growing criticism of the Emmanuel movement. At this late point
in Mitchell's career, he was in the process of assuming the presidency of the
American Neurological Association, a position initially offered to him when
the organization was founded in 1875 but that he had had to turn down because
he was too busy. Many physicians felt that clergy such as Worcester had no
business dabbling in health care, and an endorsement from Mitchell would
have gone a long way to protecting the Emmanuel movement from such criticism. One of the more acerbic attacks appeared in the *North American Review*,
wherein Dr. Allan McLane Hamilton accused Worcester and the Emmanuel
movement of being "unpardonably ignorant" and threatened that any cooperat-
ing physicians would be "taken to task by their regular Medical Societies."
Hamilton argued that the growing popularity of Christian Science depleted
traditional church congregations, especially in the northeast, and that the
Emmanuel movement was nothing more than a foolish attempt to repatriate
church members by joining in the religious doctoring game. He faulted
Christian Scientists for believing they could heal using faith, but held the
Emmanuel movement in even higher contempt for believing that clergy could
heal using crash courses in psychology. Eager to treat neurasthenia without a
full knowledge of mental illness, clergy, Hamilton warned, risked pronouncing
patients cured even though serious psychotic or manic-depressive tendencies
lay dormant, ready to explode at a terrible moment.[24]

For his part, Mitchell took an equivocal position regarding the Emmanuel
movement and its neurasthenia campaign. In his May 1908 address before the
American Neurological Association, he recognized that some victims of "lesser
neuroses" had been helped by religious mind cures and that physicians who

had never sought aid from the clergy have "missed some valuable assistance." However, he mocked the state of therapeutic spirituality in America and lambasted "Eddyism, mind cure, soul cure, [and] faith cure," as well as nonphysicians who dabbled in suggestion to relieve neurotic states such as neurasthenia. In what may or may not have been a reference to the Emmanuel movement, Mitchell claimed to know of "not less than seven of these cults." "They are alike in despising every other," he told his audience, and all were surrounded by "a vast mist of lies and suppressions of failure." In a personal letter to Dr. William Osler, a frustrated Mitchell wrote, "I am continually quoted as favourable to the Emmanuel movement. To this I say *yes* and *no*."[25] Some clergy were trained to perform therapy, he pointed out, but others were not and consequently risked aggravating health problems. Known for his personal loyalty and genial style, Mitchell could not bring himself to condemn outright Worcester's attempts to treat neurasthenia among the urban poor, but his address and private words were hardly the resounding endorsement that Worcester might have hoped for.

After two years of supporting Worcester and McComb's health campaign, Putnam eventually parted ways with the Emmanuel movement. The occasion for his change of heart was the 1908 release of the movement's handbook, *Religion and Medicine*, which he believed crossed the line between clergy wanting to *help* doctors and clergy wanting to *be* doctors. He wrote a long letter to Worcester explaining his rationale for withdrawing support. Many of his reasons paralleled critiques previously made against Christian Science, such as that the movement made reckless claims of "curing," overstated the power of mental healing, and carried a potential for unscrupulous clergy to play off emotions and exploit patients. He also questioned the "medical etiquette" of the participating clergy, especially their unfamiliarity with the referral system and their tendency to focus on mental origins of illness and ignore clear physical causes. Putnam intended his letter to be a polemic and, although he addressed it to Worcester, he sent copies to colleagues and friends, including educationalist Susan Elizabeth Blow, who relied on her own form of therapeutic spirituality to steel herself in the face of neurasthenia. "I have read your letter to Dr. Worcester with great interest," Blow informed Putnam. "It seems to me to go to the heart of every question it touches."[26]

The central question in Putnam's letter was whether the Emmanuel movement did more harm than good in eroding the line between religion and medicine already blurred by Christian Science. Putnam thought this erosion harmful, arguing that, when clergy acted as doctors, their failures discredited the medical profession as a whole. "This is what the Christian Science movement [has done]," Putnam explained, "and what the church-healing movement is doing without wishing it." He specifically mentioned Mitchell's address before the American Neurological Association, and supported the belief that, though religious healing might be useful on an ad hoc basis, it had become too big and too organized, and had gone too far.[27]

Living in an age known for celebrating the expert, Putnam defended his profession from clerical encroachment by emphasizing the need for doctors and clergy to keep their duties separate. This was the only way, he told Worcester, to "uphold the dignity of each other's profession." "A great 'profession' is a sacred thing," Putnam argued, "an outcome of the 'corporate thought' and intuition and experience of the community, a thing to be cherished and supported." Acknowledging that the clergy had an important role as the "natural critics and supporters" of doctors, he argued that they nevertheless needed to stay away from treating medical conditions unless they agreed to subject themselves "to the same sort and amount of criticism that familiarity and colleagueship demands." If clergy were to act like doctors, Putnam insisted, they must have the education, memberships, and peer review typical of the medical profession. There was room for negotiation in Putnam's mind, however, and he raised the possibility of having "an occasional conference" to discuss disorders the clergy felt equipped to treat. He even suggested the possibility, if there was enough support from the medical and pastoral communities, of establishing a "*new institution*" (a phrase he underlined in his letter), a hybrid profession to deal with the gray areas between medical and spiritual care.[28]

Hurt by criticism from mainstream medicine, the Emmanuel movement began to decline by the end of 1909, but it continued providing services for another two decades, until Worcester's retirement in 1929. Worcester and the movement incorporated emerging psychological approaches to health, including Sigmund Freud's psychoanalytical theories (of which Worcester agreed with only some), that provided therapeutic insight but were not heavily policed by scientific medicine. Starting in 1911, the movement increasingly reached out to men suffering from alcoholism and other destructive addictions, treating them in a series of group therapy meetings led by recovering alcoholics.[29] Without the full support of physicians, however, the Emmanuel movement fell short of its ultimate goal of using neurasthenia as a stepping stone to make health care the responsibility of the modern church.

The Case of Susan Elizabeth Blow

New Thought, Christian Science, and the Emmanuel movement constituted a patchwork of spiritually based mind cures available to neurasthenics around

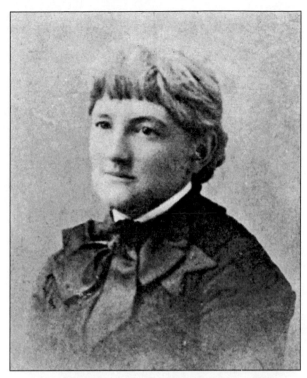

Figure 7 Susan Elizabeth Blow. A pioneer in the kindergarten movement, Blow was also a neurasthenic who developed a personal spiritual philosophy to fortify herself against her sickness. In so doing, she helped demonstrate the spiritual dimension of neurasthenia to her physician, James Jackson Putnam.

Photo courtesy of the State Historical Society of Missouri.

the turn of the century, but not all neurasthenics who recognized a spiritual dimension to their illness relied on these for guidance. Spirituality and neurasthenia, after all, were powerfully personal experiences that perceptive people could reflect upon without the guidance of self-help texts or trained religious practitioners. The case of Susan Elizabeth Blow (1843–1916), preserved in a twenty-year correspondence with her friend and neurologist, Putnam, provides an example of a woman who independently looked to religion to fortify her mind to withstand neurasthenia. "To me, life would have brought despair had it not been for the comforting relics of my Calvinism," she confided to Putnam.[30] She did not take her religion straight, but instead mixed it with scholarly ideas to develop her own spiritual philosophy. This philosophy not only proved effective therapy for her neurasthenia, but also demonstrates how neurasthenic patients could exert influence over physicians' understanding of the disease.

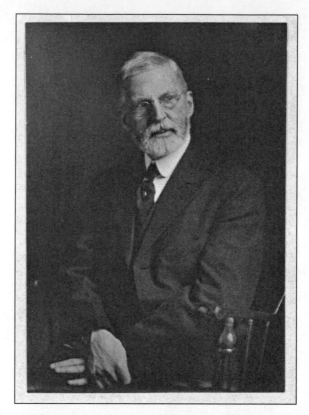

Figure 8   James Jackson Putnam, 1909. A Harvard neurologist and physician to Susan Elizabeth Blow, Putnam saw neurasthenia as a largely psychological disease, and encouraged his medical colleagues to adopt psychotherapeutic strategies to treat the condition.

Photo by Mary Cutler, 1909, courtesy of the The Harvard Medical Library in the Francis A. Countway Library of Medicine.

Born in a suburb of St. Louis into a wealthy Presbyterian family, Blow is best known today for her pioneering work in the late-nineteenth-century kindergarten movement, which sought to incorporate the teachings of German educationalist Friedrich Froebel into public school systems.[31] Working as a volunteer administrator with the St. Louis School District, she oversaw the opening of one of the nation's first public kindergarten in 1873 and began training teachers in the use of Froebel's methods. Her English translations of Froebel's work, and her own books, including *Symbolic Education* (1884) and *Educational Issues in Kindergarten* (1909), were foundational to the development of kindergartens nationwide. Neurasthenia forced her retirement from the St. Louis School District when she was forty-one and, disagreeing with those who replaced her, she left St. Louis in 1889 to live between Boston and

Cazenovia, New York, where she continued to write, give public lectures, and instruct at Teachers' College, Columbia University. At this juncture, she came under the care of Putnam, with whom she struck up a warm, philosophical, and ultimately therapeutic relationship in which each served as a sounding board for the other's ideas. "For any and all work I am able to do," she wrote Putnam in 1894, "I am in large measure indebted to your skill, fidelity, and kindness."[32]

In her gracious acknowledgement, Blow was being rather modest, as she took the leading role in regulating her own health through the development of her own philosophy. She believed that every person was composed of two parts: a soul of "infinite form," connected to a body of "finite experience." She explained to Putnam that the soul represented godly perfection, a Platonic ideal, while the body represented a person's "actual self" and earthly condition. This latter aspect of a person's identity, in her view, was imperfect—made so by personal experience, poor decisions, and "racial, national, and family inheritance." Mental and physical tension within any person was inevitable, she thought, because the ideal self almost always contrasted with the actual self. Normally this would not be a problem, as people regularly lived happy, fulfilling lives while enduring a certain amount of internal conflict and tension; however, people risked "nervous collapse and disintegration of personality" if they tried to disguise or ignored serious personal flaws, thus allowing harmful internal tension between their ideal and actual self to build unheeded. "The people I know who are threatened with collapse," she explained, "are either hiding their lesser self from the views of others and trying to seem better than they are, or else actually hiding from themselves and refusing to see something which is perpetually trying to make itself known in order to be outgrown."[33] Just as Dresser and New Thought saw illness as a call for self-help, Blow recognized her neurasthenia as evidence of a need to make adjustments to her life.

According to Blow, the key to combating neurasthenia was regulating internal tension through reflective thought. This represented a continual process of self-improvement—she often employed Froebel's educational phrase "self activity"—in which she regularly meditated upon her life and tried to become attuned to her ideal self, a focus to help her become the type of woman she felt her creator intended she be: "Having made me in his image, [he] must forever challenge me to perfection." She cited Jesus as the ultimate example of a person who achieved perfection by understanding his divine nature, and gave credit to Jesus's religious teachings for doing "more than anything else to cure my congenital defect. . . . I was born when my mother was in an unstable state and I have always had lapses into instability." The power of thought, according to Blow, could manifest physical changes within the brain to reverse what she believed were the genealogical roots of one's neurasthenia. "I need not be the victim of 'an inherited inferior brain structure,' because self-activity can modify structure," she wrote to Putnam in the summer of 1906; "I do not know where I should be without these great insights which guarantee to me my freedom and thus forever my courage."[34] Her therapeutic spiritual philosophy gave her a new lease on life, less vulnerable to the unpredictability of her neurasthenia and less reliant on physicians.

It was the rational, philosophical process behind her faith that provided much of Blow's therapeutic relief. "I am feeling the support of trust in God," she told Putnam, "but it is my intellectual conception and conviction which supports the trust." Blow's intellectual influences are not difficult to discern. She of course took Froebel very seriously, especially his emphasis on "self activity" and the need for people to "create consciously unified selves." She was well acquainted with the work of Hegel from her time in the St. Louis School District, where she worked with superintendent William T. Harris, an accomplished scholar and American translator of Hegel; indeed, her concept of moving toward an ideal self followed a sort of Hegelian dialectic. She studied, and personally knew, the Harvard pragmatists, finding her own ideas closer to those of William James than to Josiah Royce's. She kept abreast of Catholic modernism at the turn of the century, as well as James's and Henri Bergson's influences on that movement. She read the work of Sigmund Freud, and relied on Putnam, an early American follower of the Austrian neurologist, to help her understand the nuances of psychoanalytic theory. She was also acquainted with analytical philosopher Bertrand Russell and with the New Realism movement, which she considered somewhat faddish. Works on physiology and genetics by Charles Sherrington and Gregor Mendel interested her, and she seemed to have little trouble integrating them into her curative religious philosophy.[35]

As Blow's physician, Putnam recognized the therapeutic benefits of her spiritual philosophy, but he had a difficult time reconciling it with his belief in scientific medicine. Looking for answers, in the early summer of 1910 he wrote to William James, his Harvard colleague, who was convalescing in Europe and who had built a career trying to bring science and religion together. Putnam's mind was on Blow and how she dealt with her neurasthenia. "It is a pleasant life and a lovely summer's day," he observed to James, "but all these luxuries and signs of health make one feel queer in view of the fact that there are so many who are wholly ignorant of them . . . I wish you could bring home a clear philosophy and a justified religion. The 'necessary presuppositions' on which Miss Blow counts so much and which taken together with an equally 'necessary' self-activity seems to lead to such momentous conclusions, give the most comforting assurances of anything I know; but is there a flaw in them? If so, I cannot see it. And yet to feel sure! What a luxury of luxuries, and one that, fortunately, the poor can have as well as the rich."[36] Blow's spiritual certainty must have prompted this hint of envy on Putnam's part, not only because it served as the basis of her therapeutic spiritual philosophy and made his doctoring skills redundant, but because it represented an idealized, truly democratic approach to health care that relied on the faith of the masses rather than on the elite medical education of a few. His patient had affected him, and although he did not share Blow's level of faith, he nonetheless recognized a place for spirituality in the treatment of conditions such as neurasthenia.[37]

When Putnam asked James for a "clear philosophy and a justified religion," he asked the man perhaps best poised to provide both. Son of a fervent Swedenborgian, James well understood how spirituality could find its way into nearly every aspect of people's lives, from business to relationships to health. Neurasthenia was also a family trait, as he, his younger brother (novelist Henry James), and his younger sister, Alice, all suffered from debilitating depression throughout their lives. James began his academic life studying to be a physician, but he switched to psychology soon after earning his M.D. and eventually moved on to philosophy, along the way penning the discipline-defining *Principles of Psychology* (1890), *The Will to Believe, and Other Essays on Popular Philosophy* (1897), and *The Varieties of Religious Experience* (1902). Scholars since have recognized the influence James's neurasthenia had on the development of his ideas, which sought to bridge the gap between science and metaphysics.[38]

In a sense, Blow's philosophy was the culmination of her life's work and experience, as it combined the ideas of Froebel to which she had dedicated her career as a kindergarten educator, the Christian faith in which she had been reared, and the day-to-day health of her mind and body. It provided an impetus for continued learning and for discussion of new philosophical and psychological ideas, not simply because such conversations were stimulating to an intellectual woman, but also because they helped clarify her thoughts and added depth to her philosophy, a philosophy she believed central to her health. It also helped provide her life with meaning. Never married, without children, and living over a thousand miles away from St. Louis where she had made her career, had family, and would later be buried, Blow lacked many of the life-long relationships of her contemporaries. With her spiritual philosophy, however, she felt connected to the world and the nation's future. Convinced of the power of psychological "self activity" to affect changes in people, she predicted (to Putnam in 1906) that a "new birth of intellect and will" would soon take place

around the globe and spur a monumental shift in worldview: "The old conception of the universe as a mechanism was . . . from the point of view of the physi-
cist. For the last forty or fifty years we have had the universe interpreted from
the point of view of the biologist. Now it is the turn of the psychologist."[39]
Through the process of countering her neurasthenia with thought, Blow came
to see herself as a pioneer in a new psychological era that would soon define the
twentieth century.

As Blow predicted to Putnam, and Putnam predicted to Worcester, the twentieth century saw the ascendency of a relatively new therapeutic institution—
psychotherapy—that sought to harness the health benefits found in therapeutic
spirituality while preserving the professional integrity of physicians and
clergy.[40] To this end, in 1908 Putnam helped launch a series of primers,
*Psychotherapy: A Course of Reading in Sound Psychology, Sound Medicine,
and Sound Religion*, aimed at rescuing mind-cure methods from "Christian
Scientists, the New Thought people, the Faith Healers, and the thousands
and one other schools which have in common the disregard of medical science
and all the accumulative knowledge of the past."[41] In three large volumes,
published in 1908–1909, *Psychotherapy* sought to build the foundation for a
profession by bringing together seminal essays from preeminent physicians
and theologians, including the Emmanuel movement's Samuel Fallows, the
Episcopal bishop who talked to his 1907 Christmastime congregation about
using "Christian psychology" to cure neurasthenia. The arrival of European
ideas, especially the psychoanalysis of Freud (who was Putnam's guest while
visiting American in 1909), further spurred the development of psychotherapy
as a bridge between scientific medicine and therapeutic spirituality, enabling
it to far outlive the neurasthenia diagnosis to become one of the twentieth
century's most distinctive therapies.

The story of neurasthenia and therapeutic spirituality is a story of how
people struggled to define and treat illness, but men and women aching with
misery and pain did not always look inward for clues to explain their suffering.
Some searched for explanations by looking outward at the world and reflecting
on their behavior in it. Many of these people could not ignore the gendered
nature of their lives and the social and personal expectations by which they
lived as men or women. Just as spiritually inclined neurasthenics used their
illness as a prism through which to better understand their faith, those with a
heightened sense of gender used their illness as a way of understanding and
reassessing sex roles and gendered expectations in turn-of-the-century America.

Chapter 4

Neurasthenia, Health, and Gender

In his celebrated collection *The Autocrat of the Breakfast Table* (1858), Oliver Wendell Holmes observed that "man has his will—but woman has her way."[1] A simple statement, it captured the importance of one's sex in determining what a person could expect out of life in nineteenth-century genteel society. The clothes people wore, the jobs they held, the books they read, the places they occupied in the parlor: these were all indicators of gender that respectable society tended to follow. The differences in the ways men and women acted were more than mere convention; they reflected the belief that men and women were of two dissimilar, yet complementary, natures. Men, referred to as the "stronger sex," had the grit and determination to succeed in the dog-eat-dog world of politics and commerce, whereas women, known as the weaker sex, had the virtue and wisdom to sustain the nation by guiding families and households. Men provided for material need, while women served as a moral compass.[2] Catharine Beecher, a contemporary of Holmes and America's chief domestic authority during the mid-nineteenth century, reinforced the idea of men's and women's complementary natures when she explained that, although women were sometimes "made subordinate in station to men," they were compensated in other ways because "by custom and courtesy, they are always treated as superiors."[3] Men were supposedly in control, and made decisions for the benefit of women, who in turn dedicated themselves to nurturing their men and families. Ideally, all this allowed men and women to live together in harmony as friends, spouses, and parents, so long as each followed the gendered order of things.

But life is seldom ideal, and, when men and women realized that they could not live up to their expected roles, many became conflicted, despondent, and neurasthenic. Many of these men and women faulted themselves for failing to meet expectations and sought treatment just as would other neurasthenics. Some, especially those with a proclivity for introspection, wondered if the fault might lie within the nation's gendered scheme that designated social roles based on sex rather than on individual talents or interests. For these men and women, the underlying premise behind neurasthenia—that sickness arose when people lived lives for which they were unsuited—served as a heuristic springboard to critically assess sex roles and gendered expectations, in the hopes of finding the root cause of neurasthenic depression, lethargy, anxiety, and pain. Patients' resultant ideas did not develop in a vacuum but rather grew out of the interaction with friends and family, literature from the period, and caregivers.

Even though neurasthenia afflicted men and women in roughly equal numbers, each sex tended to think of its neurasthenia differently.[4] For some men, neurasthenia served as evidence that they failed in their duties as husbands and fathers and no longer possessed the powerful "will" that Holmes suggested defined manly character. Anxiety over finances, sex, and work served as seeds for neurasthenia; compensatory masculine activities and, to a lesser extent, readjustment of social roles helped combat neurasthenia and reaffirm manly identities. Women proved much more likely to trace their neurasthenia to social restraints and perceived flaws within America's gendered system. Holmes posited that women ultimately had their "way" and Catharine Beecher claimed men treated them as "superiors," but many neurasthenic women remained unconvinced of this and reevaluated their sex's social role by asking the question "What is healthy?" rather than "What is conventional?" As a whole, the presence of neurasthenia helped prod Americans into redefining their expectations for proper gendered behavior for men and women.

Neurasthenia and the Manly Will

During America's Victorian period, the ideal man possessed an indomitable will that allowed him to influence the world: voting represented his political will; control over his wife and children reflected his paternal will; and ability to earn a living signaled his economic will. Internally, the manly will ideally gave men control over their thoughts, their emotions, and their confidence. Failure to meet manly expectations signaled a potentially weak will, which drew manhood into question, thereby compounding the anxiety that led to neurasthenia. Unfortunately for American men of the time, the Victorian manly ideal often conflicted with political, social, and personal realities. Gilded Age politics were notoriously corrupt and controlled by party insiders rather than by independent men voting their consciences. Late-century market instability and the rise of the wage labor system seriously compromised men's economic self-sufficiency and ability to provide reliably for their families. Lust and impotence remained part of the human condition, as did unrestrained thoughts and emotions. For all the emphasis Americans placed on men being in *control* of their lives, at every turn appeared evidence that things were *out of control*.[5] Whereas some men took this disjuncture in stride, neurasthenics saw it as evidence of weak wills and personal failures that needed to be addressed in at least one of two ways: increased masculine activity or the adjustment of manly expectations.

The Cooper Medical Clinic

As the first medical school on the West Coast, Cooper Medical College began operating a free clinic in the 1880s as a place where people of modest means could gain medical care while students honed their skills working alongside experienced physicians. As a clinic, Cooper offered outpatient care and relied on two main forms of therapy to treat both male and female neurasthenics. The first was electrotherapy of the type advocated by George M. Beard, for which the college employed an electrotherapist to care for the clinic's faradic batteries and administer low-level current to patients. The second were drug prescriptions, often compounds incorporating bromides, quinine, or strychnine, which could be filled at the clinic dispensary at a discounted rate. As a free clinic, Cooper served much of San Francisco's working class, and its numerous neurasthenia patients illustrate how the disease indeed affected people of all classes. The clinic also kept detailed and relatively uncensored patient records for the benefit of medical students, records that today document for the historian potentially embarrassing personal problems, such as financial troubles and sexual dysfunctions, associated with neurasthenia.

Financial concerns, such as unemployment and economic setbacks, figured prominently in the neurasthenia cases of men who visited the Cooper clinic. Examples include John Reid, a sixty-one-year-old unemployed carpenter suffering from general exhaustion and weakness, symptoms that he thought might get better once he found a job and his mind had the opportunity to focus on work. Another was Hugh Clyne, a thirty-four-year-old who complained of restlessness, an inability to concentrate, a tendency to fixate on trivial things, and mental worry that grew unbearable "with loss of work." Chas Molter, a fifty-six-year-old carriage trimmer, sought help for his insomnia, constipation, and the unnerving sensation of water dripping down his head, all symptoms that began soon after he was defrauded out of a sum of money a few years before. J. O. Moore, a forty-two-year-old "traveling man" out of New York, complained of a difficulty expressing his thoughts and an impaired ability to write and make calculations, problems that he first noticed when he began worrying about business two years earlier. S. Barver, a forty-year-old unemployed fruit seller, complained of constipation, heart palpitations, disturbing dreams, feeling "weighed down," and chattering teeth, all of which he claimed started ten years earlier when "he had met with some business reverses, in consequence of which he had lost considerable money."[6]

It is unclear why Reid and Clyne were unemployed, who defrauded Molter, the nature of Moore's business problems, or how Barver lost money, but, with all these men, economic setbacks sparked unhappiness and discomfort that physicians diagnosed as neurasthenia. They stayed up at night dwelling on economic problems, the lack of sleep further impairing their mental and physical capacities. In addition, as men, their careers were central to their public identity; the rest of society knew them by the jobs they held as carpenters, carriage trimmers, business persons, and the like. In this way, unemployment or job failure not only drew into question one's manly ability to provide for the family, but also drew into question one's manly presence within the community. The neurasthenic symptoms themselves could even be seen as a loss of manly control: the men no longer had the personal will to command ambition, focus their thoughts, regulate their sleep, or even move their bowels. In essence, professional setbacks triggered what became a cascading collapse of confidence that left the men neurasthenic, despondent, and in need of help.

The neurasthenic effect of economic problems also helps explain why physicians and others had been linking neurasthenia to "overwork" since the disease's inception in 1869. Although overwork may initially appear to denote manly traits of ambition and self-sacrifice, the term also serves as a fig leaf to draw attention away from inability to keep up with the pace of work, or an incapacity for hard work—inabilities that were hardly manly traits.

In addition to suffering economic setbacks, male neurasthenics who visited the Cooper clinic often suffered from sexual dysfunctions that were downright crippling to their sense of pride and manly confidence. Frederic Curran, a twenty-nine-year-old Newfoundlander, suffered from "seminal weakness" (an involuntary discharge of semen, usually through nocturnal emission or premature ejaculation) that he blamed for his loss of ambition, general restlessness, reticence in the presence of company, and overall "stage fright" when dealing with others. Jacob Lyne, a twenty-nine-year-old Finnish gardener, considered himself in fine health until he began experiencing premature ejaculations, which then led to back pain and heart troubles; he developed an unhealthy obsession with his dysfunction, doctors noted, which drove him to

despondency. Another patient, a forty-year-old German carpenter named
M. Schlosser, went to the clinic because a decade-old case of gonorrhea had
robbed him of his "manhood" and left him impotent, which caused him to
worry himself into a neurasthenic state; for treatment, in those days before the
advent of penicillin, the attending physician gave the simple prescription to
"work hard and think less of his troubles."[7] The penis may be the most obvious
symbol of manhood, and, when men could not control its sexual function, then
any premature ejaculation and impotence made them doubt their virility and
willpower. Like financial setbacks, sexual dysfunctions had a tendency to
erode men's overall confidence and inhibit other aspects of their lives, such as
ambition, charisma, and happiness. Sexual dysfunctions also had the appearance of being entirely personal and unrelated to outside factors or influence,
which made it easier for men to place guilt for it squarely on themselves.

Masturbation represented one of the ultimate lapses of manly willpower
that characterized males' neurasthenia. Again, the Cooper clinic offers a candid
view. David Corotto, a twenty-one-year-old gardener, was troubled by poor
memory and general restlessness that he attributed to chronic masturbation;
"Patient has worried a great deal about the habit to which he is addicted," the
attending physician reported. Friends had told Corotto that masturbation was
harmful to his health, but he nonetheless indulged "uncontrollably" in the
habit; "This talk of his friends and his constant brooding over the trouble have
reduced him to the nervous condition in which he is at present," the patient
record concluded. William Oakes, a twenty-nine-year-old English janitor, came
to the clinic despondent and melancholy, claiming to have been suffering
from a "complication of nervous diseases" that caused temporary paralysis and
made him lose "control over his feelings" and laugh at inappropriate moments;
"He fears impending misfortune or evil as a punishment for masturbation prac-
ticed from the age of 15 yrs to 25 yrs," the clinic's record reported.[8] For patients
such as Corotto and Oakes, masturbation represented an inability to control
what they considered hazardous sexual urges.

During much of the nineteenth century, even the medical profession had
held the belief, shared with much of the population, that masturbation harmed
one's health. Semen supposedly contained vital energy that needed to be con-
served; masturbation represented the needless waste of this vital energy, the
loss of which many placed men at risk for the loss of intelligence, the loss of
manly willpower, and the development of neurasthenia. By the 1890s, however, the medical profession, including those at Cooper, had started shifting
attention from the loss of vital fluids as the primary health threat of masturbation toward, rather, debilitating feelings of shame caused by religious and

cultural taboo. The end result remained the same, as it was now the guilt and shame from those taboos that placed men at risk for neurasthenia.[9]

The Case of Theodore Dreiser

One of the better-documented cases of male neurasthenia was that of writer Theodore Dreiser (1871–1945), whose bout with the illness is illustrative of a perceived loss of manly willpower. Best known as one of the early twentieth century's premier writers, Dreiser established his reputation with novels, such as *Sister Carrie* (1900) and *An American Tragedy* (1925), that explored the harsh realities and challenges of modern American life and helped establish the naturalist literary movement in the nation. The son of a German immigrant, Dreiser was born in Terre Haute, Indiana, the ninth of ten children, and grew up in a family rocked by economic and emotional instability. His father was frequently unemployed, his mother struggled to make ends meet, and a strict Catholic education increased his cynicism toward the Roman Church. Although he never finished high school, Dreiser possessed a love for literature and attended Indiana University, which he left in 1890 after only a year to pursue a career in journalism. It was as a newspaper reporter in cities such as Chicago, St. Louis, Pittsburgh, and New York that Dreiser became acquainted with the darker side of American urban life, an experience that he would draw upon for his first novel, *Sister Carrie*. Although championed by fellow writer and editor Frank Norris as among the best manuscripts he had read, *Sister Carrie* drew the ire of publisher Frank Doubleday, who considered its plot of a young woman's conflict between sexuality and luxury as immoral and waged a campaign to suppress the novel's release, an action that had a deleterious effects on Dreiser's health.[10]

Today considered an American classic, *Sister Carrie* began as a commercial disappointment and Doubleday's attempt to smother the book pushed Dreiser, just over thirty, into a neurasthenic state that lasted nearly three years. Two sources give candid accounts of his illness. The first is an unfinished autobiographical story, *An Amateur Laborer*, written shortly after his recovery from the illness in 1904 but not published until 1983, decades after his death. The other source is a journal that he kept, on the advice of his physician, as a therapeutic activity while recovering from neurasthenia. Not intended for publication, it nonetheless found its way into print in 1983 as part of the volume *American Diaries, 1902–1926*. "Those who have never experienced that misfortune [of neurasthenia] cannot conceive what miseries may exist in it," Dreiser remarked at the start of "An Amateur Laborer": "I was a writer, but now my power to write was taken away from me. I could not think of anything to say or if I did I could not say it." Rather than blaming his illness on other factors, such as the poor economic showing of *Sister Carrie* or the machinations of Doubleday, Dreiser assumed responsibility for his shortcomings and repeated to himself "my fault, my fault" until the shame seemed entirely his. Dreiser's confidence sank and he lost nearly all sense of personal worth, which caused him to withdraw from society. "Sickness has apparently made a coward of me," he observed, embarrassed by this lack of manly pride.[11]

Of all his neurasthenic symptoms, the one Dreiser grieved most was his lack of mental control. "Thought failed me, reason failed me," he recorded in *An Amateur Laborer*: "I could not follow out a given chain of ideas if my life had depended on it." For a man who prided himself on putting insightful observations into lucid writing, this lack of mental control proved crippling. In his journal, he complained that his mind lacked the "power of organization" to be productive and, in the rare moments when he could accomplish some written work, he soon found himself haunted by a "disturbing sense of error" that forced him to give up. Eventually Dreiser found that "the mere thought" of writing "weakened my reasoning capacity and I at once become confused." If being intimidated by writing was not bad enough, Dreiser also experienced disturbing delusions. He found himself suffering from the "most distressing hallucinations," including the sensation that, at night, as he was trying to fall to sleep, there was someone in the room, looming over him, who would gently touch his pillow to see if he were awake. Sound sleep came rarely, as his neurasthenic mind refused to relax and instead ran wild at night, plagued by "half sensible and half disconnected thoughts" and a constant "thread of ideas" he could not muster the will to cut off. The insomnia was the worst aspect of being unable to corral his thoughts (it "seemed to be racking the soul out of me," Dreiser recalled) because the lack of sleep created a vicious cycle that left him progressively incapacitated and unable to gain the rest necessary to restore his willpower and recover control over his mind.[12]

Dreiser, like many men who visited the Cooper clinic, also had a difficult time controlling his sexual urges, which he believed aggravated his neurasthenia. "Rose at seven after having foolishly taxed myself by copulating with Mrs. D, but I could not control my desire," he wrote in his journal, obviously annoyed with himself and his early morning activities. As to why he felt the need to avoid sexual relations with his wife, Sarah (whom he called "Jug"), the most likely reason paralleled the common nineteenth-century fear concerning masturbation, that loss of semen signaled loss of vital energy. What frustrated Dreiser, though, was not simply that he had sex, but that he could not *control* his desire to. The actual sex act appeared somewhat secondary in importance to the initial sexual thoughts. "Suffered a great deal during early morning and previous evening from sexual desire which seems to affect my head," he recorded in his journal, a few days before the morning he "foolishly taxed" himself with his wife. "Managed to resist it however in so far as abstaining from copulation, but the effect of the desire was weakening."[13] Despite being able to avoid sex, desire alone was enough to frustrate him and cause the anxiety from which neurasthenia grew.

Mentally and physically exhausted, Dreiser hit rock bottom during the winter of 1902–1903. Unable to work as a writer and earn money, he could no longer support his wife and sent her away to live with her sister. Poverty forced him to pawn his watch, live in a six-foot-by-eight-foot tenement room, eat food he found on the street, and shed weight until his six-foot frame supported only 130 pounds. Even attempts to find work as a manual laborer failed, as his physical frailty and natural bookishness discouraged employers from hiring him. "The grimness of this to me was that it was the climax of a series of incidents that had been constantly revealing to me the wretchedness and inadequacy of my character," he explained in *An Amateur Laborer*. Utterly despondent, he feared that neurasthenia would be the end of him and he would never be able to recover control over his mental capacities again: "Then I am doomed to it, forever. Oh dreadful ending."[14]

Dreiser's older brother, Paul, rescued him from neurasthenic poverty and despair when the two met quite by accident on the streets of New York City. Recognizing his brother needed help, Paul, a successful songwriter, insisted on sending him to a sanitarium to recover. Sparing no expense, he shuttled Dreiser off to Muldoon's Farm, a rehabilitation community in White Plains, New York, run by William Muldoon, an ex-champion wrestler turned personal trainer. Muldoon called his health farm a "human repair shop" and promised to work his clients, almost exclusively men and many neurasthenic, back into top physical and mental shape, an experience Dreiser recounted in his short story "Scared Back to Nature." The strong and agile Muldoon exuded a "dominating presence," according to the author, and toughened his worn-out clients by putting them through a barrage of physical activity and verbal abuse. During exercises, Muldoon employed his booming voice to taunt his patients and used his superior conditioning to belittle what strength and agility they brought to his camp. "'Hurry up now! Faster! Put the ball back to me. Do you want it all day? What are you standing there for?'" Muldoon mocked while pelting men— his patients—in the neck and chest with three-pound medicine balls to encourage activity. Activities such as this, Dreiser sensed, took from the men their last shreds of dignity. From Dreiser's perspective, Muldoon made it his job to physically and mentally control his patients as tightly as possible; even during meals he bullied people, ordering one man to eat unwanted carrots and forbidding another from having a second glass of buttermilk.[15]

Sure enough, Muldoon's bullying began to have a beneficial effect, as Dreiser stopped thinking about his personal problems, built up his agility and strength, and began to feel better. Muldoon explained to Dreiser that the secret to his success treating neurasthenia was in creating an environment wherein men might rest their overtaxed minds long enough to recover. His rough manner was nothing more than "a method of wrestling a man's mental control from him in order to increase his mental energy. If his will has nothing to do with the arrangements of his day, his mind is much more likely to contemplate nature and to rest."[16] By dictating what time patients awoke, what time they slept, how much they ate, how hard they exercised, and even the way they bathed, Muldoon sought to lift the burdens of thought and decision-making from neurasthenic men overwhelmed by their lives and responsibilities. Although their bodies were put to work, their minds were allowed to rest and their willpower replenished, so that when they left Muldoon's they possessed just enough manly will to control their thoughts and sleep habits and to slowly reintegrate themselves into society as engaged, productive men.

In many ways, Muldoon's Farm served as a masculine work-cure version of Mitchell's rest cure, a neurasthenia treatment intended mainly for women. Just as Muldoon relied on his strong personality to bully his patients into acquiescence, Mitchell insisted the rest cure be administered by a doctor in possession of "a firm and steady will" that could "insure belief in his opinions and obedience to his decrees."[17] Both Muldoon and Mitchell relied on tightly controlling their patients' diet, exercise (or lack thereof, in the case of the rest cure), and other daily functions. In addition, both required in-patient care apart from families and jobs that were presumably the sources of their neurasthenic anxiety in the first place. The obvious difference between Muldoon's work cure and Mitchell's rest cure, of course, is that while Muldoon cultivated a hypermasculine environment of rigorous exercise, verbal taunting, and violent intimidation, Mitchell relied on a hyperfeminized environment of undisturbed bed rest, muscle massages, and patriarchal instruction. One catered to the male neurasthenics, the other to the female neurasthenics, but both sought to create highly structured environments wherein the mind could rest and rejuvenate.

Redefining the Manly Ideal

Not everyone agreed with Muldoon that the best way to cure men's neurasthenia was through a masculine work cure. Some people faulted American manly ideals as unrealistic and destined to break men who tried to achieve them. In 1910, *The American Magazine* published "The Autobiography of a Neurasthenic," an anonymous account of an overworked lawyer's neurasthenic breakdown that challenged popularly held ideas regarding what constituted manly behavior. One day, without apparent cause, the narrator, a "great, strapping, full-bodied man," began crying uncontrollably. Self-conscious of his "lack of 'manliness'" and paralyzed by self-doubt, he found himself in a "constant state of terror" that he felt compelled to hide, out of embarrassment. Few people knew of his condition, and even the prospect of confiding to his wife was untenable for him: "Anything else I could tell her—but not that." He had always fulfilled his duties as husband and father, but now feared he might become unable to provide for his family or head it: the "shame of my sickness was bound up in the thought of [my wife] and the children." The narrator was evidently not alone in feeling insecure in his manliness, as friends emerged to help console him by confessing their own personal insecurities. "I would argue to myself," a fellow neurasthenic told him, "that I was a failure as a man and as a husband and father."[18] The rest of the story detailed the narrator's longing for sympathy, his thoughts of suicide (made worse by witnessing an unemployed man jump off a bridge), and his search for treatment, a search that involved general practitioners, medical specialists, hypnotists, a self-administered meditative mind cure, gymnasium workouts, and therapeutic baths.

Relief finally came when he chose to opt out of competitive professional life and spend more time with friends and family. He realized that he had fooled himself into thinking that he worked hard for his family, when in fact his efforts only served to satisfy his self-absorption. "I used to worry about the career of my boy. I wanted him to become a great lawyer," the narrator explained. "Now I believe I should be glad if he were to decide to become a farmer. I dread the dangers of his striving for success; I want him instead to keep healthy and happy and to enjoy himself as he goes along."[19] Sickness led the reflective author of "Autobiography of a Neurasthenic" to realize that a man did not have to use workplace success to prove himself a dutiful husband and father; after all, it was *over-dedication* to work that had caused the neurasthenia that risked severing his relationship with his family. Money and recognition were important, the narrator acknowledged, but his bout with neurasthenia demonstrated that they meant nothing without one's health and family. The lesson learned was that sometimes a man had to muster the gumption to step out of the high-pressured career track and redefine his familial role from hard-working provider to ever-present supporter.

In their attempts to alleviate men's neurasthenia, both Muldoon and the author of "Autobiography of a Neurasthenic" sought to redefine manliness.

As an ideal, manliness carried expectations that few men could live up to, and instances of unemployment, timidity, lack of concentration, insomnia, and lack of sexual control risked being interpreted a failure of manly will, which threatened to feminize men. "I thought at one time, when I was about your age, that nerves, as well as stomachs, belonged to cows and sick women," Alfred I. du Pont of gunpowder and chemical fame wrote to Frank L. Connable, his general manager, while du Pont was resting his nerves in rugged South Dakota during the late summer of 1906; "Unfortunately, I find out now that I have both."[20]

If neurasthenic men were to overcome the shame associated with their condition, they had to resolve the tensions inherent within the manly ideal. Muldoon sought to do this by deemphasizing manly self-control and responsibility, and emphasizing masculine physicality and aggressiveness; his masculine activities ostensibly let men's minds rest, but they also helped counteract the potentially feminizing aspects of male neurasthenia by reminding men that they still were, literally, the stronger sex capable of surviving the world's harsh realities. Alternatively, rather than move toward masculinity, the narrator of "The Autobiography of a Neurasthenic" suggested men revise their manly responsibilities to divest themselves from unhealthy dedication to work and reinvest themselves into nurturing and caring for their families, thereby reducing men's workplace anxiety while increasing the healthy emotional support of loved ones.

Neurasthenia and Women's Roles

The fatigue, indecisiveness, and emotionality associated with neurasthenia were feminized traits that encouraged people such as du Pont to think of neurasthenia as a women's disease. For years, the quintessential neurasthenic was popularly seen as an upper-class woman who used her illness as an excuse to avoid unwanted engagements, and who followed leisurely diversions when not recuperating at home, à la Hoppin's *Fashionable Sufferer*. She was neurasthenic because she could afford to be, and could rest during the day while other women were busy raising families and keeping house. While some neurasthenics most likely fit this mold and saw in the condition an opportunity to luxuriate, many honestly traced their illness to what they considered unhealthy domestic responsibilities. What, exactly, constituted unhealthy responsibilities tended to differ from woman to woman, however. Similarities between neurasthenic women existed, though, and examining the cases of three neurasthenic patients of Mitchell—Amelia Gere Mason, Sarah Butler Wister, and Charlotte Perkins Gilman—reveals that domesticity could be unhealthy and that neurasthenia served as a powerful motivator for women to revamp their domestic and social responsibilities and insist on greater freedom in the "way" (to use Holmes's term) they lived their lives.[21]

The Case of Amelia Gere Mason (1831–1923)

Born Amelia Ruth Gere in 1831 in Northampton, Massachusetts, Mason moved west with her family, as a young girl, to Chicago, a city that more or less remained her home until her death in 1923. After earning her degree in music with a specialty in singing from Mount Holyoke College in 1851, she served as principal of a private school and taught classics until neurasthenia struck and her health failed, forcing her to withdraw from teaching and administration. Later, she resumed her career as a music tutor, literary critic, essayist, and historian. Mason's neurasthenia came and went in cycles, allowing her to teach and write while she was healthy, but forcing her into seclusion—often to a place outside the city—while ill. Marriage did not seem to have been a high priority for Mason, as she waited until she was forty-one before wedding entrepreneur Alverin Armington Mason (1822–1904) in 1872. They had no children.[22]

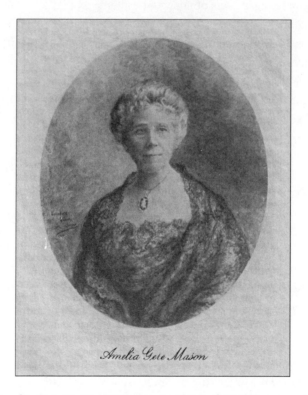

Figure 9   Amelia Gere Mason, 1904. A neurasthenic from Chicago, and a patient of S. Weir Mitchell, Mason saw her sickness as the product of a modern world that lacked inspiration. She thought it women's responsibility to rescue American culture and infuse it with unifying, inspirational sentiment.

Portrait by Elizabeth Gowdy Baker, 1904, from Amelia Ruth Gere Mason, *Memories of a Friend* [Chicago: Laurence C. Woodworth, 1918], 89.

Mason took advantage of the culture that Chicago offered a woman of comfortable means. She visited exhibitions and kept abreast of the art world by reading the cutting-edge journal *The New Path* and the more mainstream *Fortnightly*. She found herself part of a community of culturally minded women that revolved around Kate Newell Doggett, an avid botanist, skilled dancer, and vice-president of the National Woman Suffrage Association. These women devoured Charles Dickens, William Makepeace Thackeray, George Eliot, and Nathaniel Hawthorne; considered Ralph Waldo Emerson their "sage and philosopher"; religiously read *The Nation*; and valued James Russell Lowell and the *Atlantic* group as a "national treasure." By the late 1860s, she and her friends carried on, as Mason recalled, an "indefatigable search for everything that could throw a ray of light on what was going on in the world of art and intellect."[23] Without children or a large household to tend, she made culture and ideas the manna on which she lived.

In 1873, Doggett's circle, inspired by Matthew Arnold's *Culture and Anarchy* (1869) and John Stuart Mill's *The Subjection of Women* (1869), had evolved into The Fortnightly, a formal club that met in the tradition of the French salons and dedicated itself to the intellectual and cultural development of women. The similarity between The Fortnightly and French salons was no coincidence, as Chicago was then home to the glamorous Madame d'Hericourt, a former salon hostess in exile from France who frequently gave lectures on literature, society, politics, and philosophy. The legacy of European salons, especially women's role in them, left an indelible mark on Mason, who later traveled to Europe to research the history of the French salons and in 1891 published the well-received (and still widely available) work of biography and philosophy, *The Women of the French Salons*.[24]

Mason attributed her neurasthenia to a combination of factors, including unbridled thought, excessive activity, and the need to care for her husband. "Intellectual enthusiasms are wearing," she complained to Mitchell, her friend and physician; "thinking too severely exhausts me." She had explosions of activity in which she penned essays (on literature, music, and society), published books on the history of women, presented papers at society meetings, read the latest novels, and kept up with friends. But inevitably her motivation would collapse under a demanding schedule. "I wish to do twenty things at once, hence, I am idle," she explained to Mitchell. With her energy exhausted, her thoughts veered toward despondency, especially during the holiday season, when her life lacked inspiration, joy, and hope. "I stay here," she somberly wrote during a Chicago winter, "because it is a very good place to die in. There is so little that is interesting to leave." The need to nurse her sick husband, who suffered from vertigo and crippling falls, also weighed heavily on her mind. "Everything falls on my weak shoulders," she lamented; "I give out but get up and stumble on ... the Sword of Damocles hangs always over my head." Following her husband's death, Mason felt even greater loneliness and isolation. "The flowers and souvenirs scattered about my room tell me that I am not forgotten," she remarked to Mitchell a few days after Christmas, "but I feel on the outside of things and it is chilly."[25]

At the root of Mason's illness was a lack of inspiration, which she believed reflected a much larger national crisis taking place in turn-of-the-century America. The United States, she argued, had become coldly modern and overly dedicated to business and material things at the expense of romanticism, creativity, and the cultural elements that brought communities together into an organic whole. "This clear, bright, modern light—I don't like it. No perspective, no high sentiment of the permanent sort, no imagination!" she wrote to Mitchell in 1900.[26] Mason traced this problem back to men, who were constantly engaged in a "race for money," always thinking of the "utilitarian side of life," and unwilling to dedicate their talent to the arts, which might serve as the bedrock of society. As a relatively young nation, America lacked a deep-rooted national culture and consequently seemed to Mason to be unequipped to withstand inevitable challenges. Late nineteenth-century events seemed to support Mason's fears, as the Civil War gave way to violent labor disputes, such as the Great Railroad Strike of 1877, the Haymarket Square Riot of 1886, and the Pullman Strike of 1894. Also, the rise of lynching in the South during the 1890s and the influx of millions of new immigrants from Eastern Europe and the Mediterranean revealed deep racial and ethnic divisions. At the turn of the twentieth century, Mason believed that America was in particular need of the moral, stabilizing influence of artistic and literary culture. With men dedicating themselves to business, "This work was clearly to fall upon women," she claimed, "if done at all."[27]

Representative of Mason's hope that women could help strengthen American culture was her work of intellectual history and philosophy, *The Women of the French Salons*. The product of seven years of European archival research and personal interviews, the book sought to record the contributions made by upper-class French women to their nation's culture and stability during the nineteenth century by hosting salons and acting as patrons of art and thought. Mason's study also called for American women to mobilize in defense of their own national culture, which she thought was weakened by shallow materialism perpetuated by business-minded men. "It is in France that we find the forerunners of the intelligent, self-poised, clear-sighted, independent modern woman," her preface observed.[28] With this book, Mason attempted to preserve the tradition of woman as intellectual that she had first encountered a quarter-century earlier with Madame d'Hericourt, Kate Newell Doggett, and The Fortnightly club. Her opus responded to those who claimed that women best served their nation by remaining healthy and bearing children—a belief that categorically excluded the neurasthenic and childless Mason. Instead, she celebrated the potential for educated women of all ages, married and unmarried, with or without children, sick or healthy, to strengthen their nation through cultural and intellectual endeavors.

Mason also recognized that, to improve their health, women needed to be able to follow personal interests, even if doing so led to careers traditionally dominated by men and broke the convention of men and women keeping to separate spheres. She realized that many people disagreed, not the least among whom was Mitchell, her own physician, who claimed that such behavior not only risked overexertion and sickness but also risked spoiling women's feminine virtue—their "true attractiveness"—thereby making them less fit to be a man's "friendly lover." For Mitchell, that is, women best served society as complements to men, supporting their husbands and families, roles that he believed were threatened when women competed with men academically or professionally.[29]

During an epistolary exchange in which Mitchell claimed that women physicians lacked "poetic femininity," Mason defended her position and sharply reprimanded her doctor: "Why should a woman with a capacity for certain things quite legitimate and honorable, spend her life in poverty and distasteful toil because men think the things she likes and can do, unpoetic, or rather why do men think the practical embodiment of the ministering angel unpoetic? Is it less poetic to prescribe for the sick than to nurse them, or to make bread, or to sew?"[30] Mason's participation in Doggett's salon had emboldened her faith in women's intellectual and social abilities. She recognized a place in medicine for women's sympathetic ("poetic") character, a conviction shared by medical pioneer Elizabeth Blackwell and a generation of other nineteenth-century female physicians.[31] Also, by linking professional restrictions and social prejudice faced by women with the "poverty and distasteful toil" in which they often found themselves, Mason recognized how women were challenged by combined factors, including economics, ostracism, and patriarchy: "I sympathize with the poor girls who are forced to choose between two paths of misery—doing something they don't like, or living under the ban of man's disapproval . . . under penalty of social annihilation—what sort of choice is it?"[32] Unless society adjusted its attitude toward allowing women greater access to careers outside the home, Mason worried that those who disliked traditional domestic work were ultimately doomed to become neurasthenic, either by the depression of a lifetime of dull labor or by the anxiety caused by social condemnation.

Feeling trapped in an unimaginative nation and cognizant of the social restrictions women faced in following their interests beyond the conventional, Mason did not place her hopes on the establishment of women's legal rights so much as on getting men to begin treating women with respect and deference. A conservative at heart, she believed in a gendered social order and was not in favor of women's suffrage, or of any sort of universal equality. "The barrier [preventing equality] is a natural, not an artificial one," she observed to Mitchell. "Equality pure and simple is a dream. It has never existed and in the nature of things never can exist." The problem lay with men, including Mitchell himself, Mason argued, who overestimate women's "humility under masculine despotism": "A woman loves strength, but not a despotic assertion of it. She may love to yield, because she prefers some other will to her own, but never to be made to yield." Mason insisted that choice, rather than duty, should be the basis for women's decisions; to think otherwise, she informed Mitchell, was a "popular fallacy" that "the coming woman will dissipate." If men failed to create a cohesive national culture, then they needed to move aside for women to do so, and if a woman found happiness by turning her talents toward the professions, then men should honor that. "I don't like all of the changes in attitude of women," Mason wrote to Mitchell in 1912, when she was in her eighties, "but I like less the old attitude *toward* them, which stamped them with inferiority in spite of a pretense of chivalry."[33] In spirit, Mason embraced the gendered ideal put forward by Holmes and Beecher, but in practice, she realized, it wore down women, who needed more forcefully to assert their prerogative to live the way they thought necessary.

The Case of Sarah Butler Wister (1835–1908)

Sarah Butler Wister was another accomplished neurasthenic patient and correspondent of Mitchell. Born in 1835, she was of the same generation as Mason but identified more closely with homemaking. It was these things—taking care of husband, son, and large family estate—that Wister cherished, but that she nonetheless believed lay at the root of her neurasthenia. Where Mason's relationship with Mitchell evolved from that of a patient into that of a friendly intellectual partnership, Wister and Mitchell were cousins as well as patient and doctor. Consequently their letters typically dealt with family matters more often

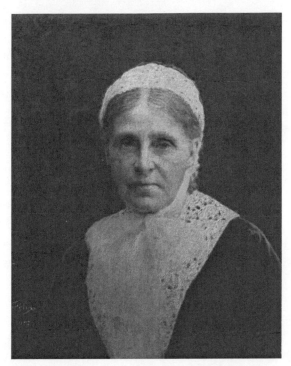

Figure 10   Sarah Butler Wister, 1907. In charge of a large family estate, Wister blamed her neurasthenia on her excessive responsibilities to keep her home running smoothly. She ended up finding a semblance of health by taking restful vacations.

The Historical Society of Pennsylvania, Society Portrait Collection.

than with health. Yet each looked to the other for professional aid: Mitchell relied on Wister as an informal editor of his novels and, according to a biographer, as the model for several of his heroines, while Wister relied on Mitchell for medical advice.[34]

Growing up, Wister was the oldest daughter in a family that was troubled from the start. Her father, Pierce Butler, owned Georgia plantations and was one of the largest slaveholders of the antebellum period. Her mother, the famous English actress Fanny Kemble, was an ardent abolitionist who claimed that she did not know the source of her husband's income until after they had married, and who wrote treatises against slavery throughout the late 1830s, the most famous being *Journal of a Residence on a Georgian Plantation,* published during the Civil War. Unwilling to live with her slave-holding husband and to abide by his increasingly abusive ways, Kemble left for London in 1845 to rekindle an acting career. She returned to America three years later to defend herself unsuccessfully against divorce when Butler sued on grounds of abandonment. Sarah and her sister Frances stayed in the custody of their father. Despite her mother's flight to London and subsequent divorce, the young Sarah Wister grew to appreciate her mother's abolitionism and artistic interests.[35]

Wister's adult life both rejected and resembled that of her mother. She married Dr. Owen Jones Wister, a Quaker, in 1859, and had one son, Owen Jr. She and her family lived at Butler Place, her father's eighty-two-acre estate in Philadelphia, where she took her housekeeping and mothering duties seriously until her death in 1908. Wister kept up her mother's artistic tradition by writing poetry and essays and by entertaining literary figures such as William Dean Howells, Henry James, and English poet Matthew Arnold.[36] Befitting a woman who grew up with ideologically opposed parents, Wister tended to strike a balance in her friendships and politics. One of her closest confidantes since childhood was Mitchell, with whom she traded family gossip and exchanged emotional support. Another close friend was Agnes Irwin, coeditor with Wister of a centennial volume, *Worthy Women of Our First Century* (1877), and eventually the dean of Radcliffe College. Wister divided her reading between the progressive *The Nation* and Herbert Welsh's anti-imperialist *City and State*.[37]

Poor health and feelings of isolation dogged Wister most of her life, as she found herself surrounded by nervous sickness within her own family. Her husband suffered from neurasthenia for much of his life, her son experienced a nervous breakdown in 1884, and her sister-in-law (also named Sarah) consistently suffered from what Wister disparagingly called a "demi-malade imaginaire."[38] Looking back on her life, Wister recalled that her most profound problems began when she was only fifteen and had developed a morbid desire for death, which she described as the "longest, strongest wish of my life." By the 1860s, she began to experience chronic insomnia, which lasted more than thirty years, stopping temporarily around the time of her husband's death in 1896 but beginning again after her son's marriage in 1898. "I am profoundly convinced that . . . each soul must struggle through the bitter floods alone," Wister confided to Mitchell. "The doubts, the despairs, play their parts in the scheme, whatever it may be." Despite this stoicism, Wister relied heavily on personal relationships for peace of mind and stability. While in Europe with her mother in the summer of 1870, she experienced a period of extreme anxiety when faced with the marriage of her closest childhood friend, Jeannie Field Musgrove. The loss of friends and family aggravated her neurasthenia, causing incapacitating neck and back pain. "I felt a terrible nervous jab," Wister reported to Mitchell upon hearing of the death of family friend and prominent Philadelphia physician Jacob DaCosta. "I was really helpless. I [couldn't] bear the fatigue of keeping house."[39]

Even when faced with a good friend's death, Wister could not put house-keeping out of her mind. She both resented it as a chore and cherished it as a responsibility.[40] She explained to Mitchell how she became "infuriated" when forced to set down an engrossing book to attend to housework, an activity she found required "immense attention." Yet when she employed the services of an assistant to help relieve the demands of domestic work, she found herself overcompensating with a "mad gallop for errands [and] chores" that occupied her until late into the evening, by which time she was too tired to read a book or write a letter.[41] Keeping house exacerbated Wister's nervous disposition. Her first test came in 1861 while she supervised the spring cleaning of the sizeable Butler Place. Despite precautions, workers' attempts to whitewash and clean the chimneys resulted in a fiasco that filled the house with "an avalanche of soot." Directing hired help frustrated her completely. "The servants, despite their lofty pretension," Wister wrote in her journal, "are just as incompetent as if they had never lived in a house in their life, & so inattentive that they forget your orders while you are speaking & disobey them under your eyes." Reliant on servants with whom she had a difficult relationship, and painfully aware of the potential pitfalls of running a large estate, she found the strain of her responsibilities manifesting itself in her body and mind. "I have not the physical strength for it nor the moral serenity," she admitted during that first fateful seasonal cleaning. In 1881, after twenty years of "household worry," Wister's health finally gave out in what she later described as a "terrible nervous break-down" followed by two years of melancholia. She blamed housekeeping, yet she could not put it aside, and upon recovery she continued to supervise the estate's upkeep for another twenty years.[42]

Given her compulsion to overwork, Wister found solace in taking pre-scribed breaks that permitted periods of industriousness while offering relax-ation and recuperation.[43] The idea of taking a break from stressful work was not new to her; after all, Mitchell, her cousin, had become a minor celebrity for advising people to take more holidays, and her son, Owen Jr., overcame his own bout of neurasthenia by traveling to the West in 1885, an experience he avidly wrote his mother about and used as the basis of his widely popular cowboy novel, *The Virginian* (1902).[44] Without prescribed breaks, relaxing did not seem possible for Wister, especially during the final years of her husband's life when he was particularly demanding of her attention. As her doctor, Mitchell advised her to dedicate time every day to practice painting watercolor landscapes. Unsure if she had much talent, Wister set out to test her abilities and ended up spending two to three hours every morning outdoors by herself, working on her art during the summer of 1893. She found it an invigorating experience, as it forced her to stay in the fresh air "twice as much as usual" and gave her "tranquility of mind." "For this," she enthusiastically wrote to Mitchell, "I am your willing debtor."[45]

Realizing the importance of setting aside time for herself marked Wister's growing understanding that modern women needed time off from their family duties to reach their full potential. During a discussion in 1895 as to why women so rarely did "first-rate work in art or literature," Wister argued to Mitchell that the answer lay in their overwhelming domestic responsibilities and their lack of personal time. It was impossible for women to "protect themselves from interruptions—the constant necessity of 'side tracking,'" while looking after the home and all those within. French novelist George Sand, Wister pointed out, did her best work when she lived "à la Bohème without domestic ties or cares" so she could rigidly enforce her "daily privilege of solitude while writing." Wister also looked to English novelist George Eliot, who produced her best work only after her companion, the writer George Lewes, was at hand to "relieve her of every trivial task."[46] The example of Wister's mother, Fanny Kemble, who found it impossible to play at once the roles of traditional wife and successful actress, may have also helped Wister believe in the incompatibility of complete dedication to the family and to artistic excellence. If women were to make the healthy decision to develop their individual talents and identities, she felt they needed to take the potentially unorthodox step of safeguarding personal time, even if it meant reducing domestic duties.[47]

After the death of her husband, Wister spent the spring and summer in a resort in rural Summerville, South Carolina, where she found the environment she needed to revitalize her ailing mind and body. A masseuse who traveled around town on a bicycle was on hand to ease her back pains but, most important, she had solitude. "I never had a more peaceful Easter tide," she recalled. She was "alone, quite alone for the hotel was empty save for one quiet family and two invisible invalids." Away from the burdens, bustle, and memories of Butler Place, Wister could contemplate her widowhood and her son's impending marriage without distraction. In time, she met local people and developed a sense of community that helped alleviate some of her nervousness as she realized that her new acquaintances had the same family worries she did. "I was calming and fortifying my soul and, for the first time with any sort of success, [trying] to reconstruct my remnant of life," she explained to Mitchell. She did not rely exclusively on Summerville for relaxation; on other occasions, she visited Homestead Hot Springs in Virginia, where she received regular courses of baths and treatments that created a "general inability and disinclination for the least mental exertion." The prescribed necessity for physical, mental, and emotional relaxation essentially gave her permission to focus on her own needs rather than those of her family and home.[48] Importantly, she did this without having to reject her life as a homemaker. These breaks, whether a few hours of morning painting or a few months of vacation, also allowed Wister to recognize the personal sacrifices women made as wives and mothers. Thus, Wister was in effect able to follow her mother and experience freedom as an independent woman without having to make her mother's sacrifice of family ties in the process.

The Case of Charlotte Perkins Gilman (1860–1935)

Writer and intellectual Charlotte Perkins Gilman also realized the link between women's domestic duties and neurasthenia. Yet rather than provide recuperative breaks from housework, such as Wister took, Gilman believed society needed to redefine and modernize housework to make it healthier for women. She sought to prove social conservatives such as Mitchell wrong, and her own egalitarian beliefs right, by affixing blame for neurasthenia on America's patriarchal society and its primitive system of household labor, rather than on any inherent weakness in women.[49] She represented, essentially, the "coming woman" that fellow neurasthenic Mason thought would reverse many traditional attitudes toward women held by people such as Mitchell.

Born in 1860, Gilman was a generation younger than Mason, Wister, and Mitchell. Like Wister, she came from a broken home; her father, Frederick Beecher Perkins, abandoned the family and left his wife, Mary, his son, Thomas, and his daughter, Charlotte, without a steady source of income. Economic straits forced Gilman's mother (the most "passionately domestic of home-worshipping wives") to move with the children from relative to relative nearly twenty times before settling in Providence, Rhode Island. Gilman remembered her mother as emotionally distant, a characteristic that Gilman assumed grew from a desire on her mother's part to instill emotional resiliency to protect her children from being hurt as her estranged husband had hurt her.[50] The family problems, economic hardships, and unfulfilled relationships of Gilman's childhood foreshadowed similar problems that would arise later in her struggle with neurasthenia.

Geared toward a life of independence since girlhood, she was twenty-three when she married painter Charles Walter Stetson and, less than a year later, had her only child, Katharine. Tragedy ensued. With pregnancy came a severe depression that worsened after she gave birth. Looking back decades later,

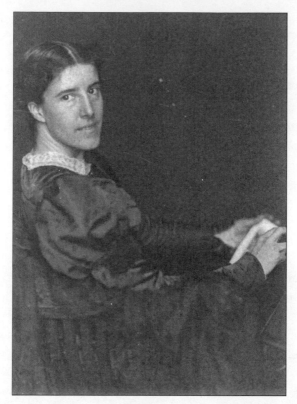

Figure 11   Charlotte Perkins Gilman, ca. 1900. An author, economist, and social activist, Perkins underwent a harrowing experience with Weir Mitchell's rest cure, eventually concluding that women became neurasthenic not because they tried to do too much, but because they were not allowed to do enough.

Photo by Francis Benjamin Johnston, ca. 1900. Image from Frances Benjamin Johnston Collection, the Library of Congress.

Gilman described her condition as "dragging weariness miles below zero. Absolute incapacity. Absolute misery." Whereas she had been "ceaselessly industrious" before marriage, her illness made her incapable of anything other than crying helplessly on the sofa. Nursing her baby was loveless and painful. "The tears ran down on my breast," she recalled; "Nothing was more utterly bitter than this, that even motherhood brought no joy." All that she once found pleasurable—reading, writing, and painting—no longer held meaning for her. On the advice of a doctor, she quickly weaned her baby, placed her in the care of her mother, and in 1886 left by train to stay the winter with friends in Pasadena, California, in the hope that the change in environment would help her recuperate.[51]

Gilman's California vacation was a success. Although she brought along a supply of tonics and sedatives, she found that she felt better as soon as the train started moving west, away from her family. En route to Pasadena, she visited her brother in Utah where she enjoyed herself riding in the mountains and attending a lively party of rowdy cowboys. In California she stayed with the family of her childhood friend Grace Channing; surrounded by fresh air, scenic mountains, friendly society, and plenty of active sports, Gilman quickly recovered and regained her vigor and energy. "Hope came back, love came back, I was eager to get home to husband and child, life was bright again."[52]

As soon as she returned to her family in Providence, however, she fell back into the funk that she thought was conquered. This latest bout of neurasthenia brought her to an agonizing realization: she was healthy while away and sick while at home. Faced with the prospect of having to choose between life as a mother and wife or her personal health, she fell into "utter prostration . . . inner misery . . . [and] ceaseless tears." For a time she relied on the patent medicine Essence of Oats, but found in it only temporary relief. Having hit rock bottom, Gilman attracted the attention of a family friend who offered to pay for a consultation with Mitchell, the nation's foremost specialist on neurasthenia.[53]

Gilman's ill-fated encounter with Mitchell has helped earn the doctor a notorious reputation among scholars today, and earned her the reputation of being a victim of patriarchal medicine. Thinking that Mitchell might find an account of her illness useful, Gilman made a case history of herself in preparation for their meeting. Rather than being pleased, Mitchell shocked her by dismissing her effort as an act of self-conceit. Their relationship deteriorated from there. In her autobiography, Gilman claimed that Mitchell never understood her condition because she was neither of the two types of patients he normally treated: neurasthenic businessmen "exhausted from too much work" and neurasthenic society women "exhausted from too much play." A hasty judgment on Gilman's part, the statement was revealing of the difficulty she and Mitchell had in relating to each other. Mitchell diagnosed her with neurasthenia and treated her with his trademark rest cure, which she took with "utmost confidence." After supervising a month of enforced bed rest, sponge baths, and massages, Mitchell declared Gilman cured and discharged her with this infamous prescription: "Live as domestic a life as possible. Have your child with you all the time. . . . Lie down an hour after each meal. Have but two hours' intellectual life a day. And never touch pen, brush, or pencil as long as you live."[54]

For months, Gilman closely followed Mitchell's orders and severely cut down on her intellectual activity. Rather than recovering, however, she found herself "perilously near" to losing her mind. She took to hiding in a closet and playing with a rag doll. "The mental agony grew so unbearable," she later recalled, "that I would sit blankly moving my head from side to side—to get out from under the pain." Upon recovery, she used this experience and its mental torture as the basis for her harrowing short story "The Yellow Wallpaper" (1892), whose protagonist is slowly driven insane by the rest cure's intellectual and social isolation.[55]

Gilman's destructive attempt to follow Mitchell's order to "live as domestic of a life as possible" affirmed the conclusion she had come to earlier when she returned from California: playing the conventional role of wife and mother made her sick. Despite these presumed roots of her suffering, she never *rejected* the idea of marriage and family; indeed, she married George Gilman six years after divorcing Stetson and always cherished her daughter, Katharine. She objected instead to the division of labor in the typical family that forced mothers and wives to follow antiquated and inefficient work schedules that exhausted women and made them nervous wrecks. Her 1893 short story "Through This" conveyed the hectic pace of a woman consumed by housework. Told in the first person, the story presented a housewife who woke before sunrise, inspired with domestic purpose: "I live. I can help. Here close at hand lie the sweet home duties through which my life shall touch others! Through this man made happier and stronger by my living; through these rosy babies sleeping here in the growing light; through this small, sweet, well-ordered home whose restful influence shall touch all comers; through me too, perhaps . . . I must get up, or this bright purpose fades."[56] The rest of her day was a breathless dash to light stoves, cook, set tables, take care of children, coo over her husband, shop, sew, clean, arrange for household repairs, and catch some sleep as the sun sets—all with no thought of herself and only passing recognition of the world outside her home. She was a paragon of domesticity and she kept busy to avoid having to face the fact that she lived vicariously through her husband and children and lacked an independent identity of her own. She was a middle-class version of Sarah Butler Wister before the breakdown.

The question of how to make domestic labor more responsive to women's psychological and physical health influenced much of Gilman's literary work. In "Making a Change" (1911), she told the story of Julia Gordins, a young woman who gave up her happy single life as a music teacher for an unhappy marriage, a colicky baby, and a mother-in-law who continually questioned Julia's parenting skills. Family tensions rose and Julia, feeling a failure as both a wife and a mother, became depressed and attempted suicide by turning on the gas in her room. The older Mrs. Gordins heroically rescued her by climbing through the transom, whereupon she intuitively recognized her daughter-in-law's plight and immediately became empathetic. "I understand. I *understand*," Mrs. Gordins comforted Julia, "I've got the *loveliest* plan to tell you about! We *are* going to make a change!"[57]

Just as Alexander the Great decisively met the challenge of the Gordian knot with a slice of his sword, Mrs. Gordins and Julia cut family tensions by redefining labor responsibilities to reflect more closely each woman's interests and abilities. Mrs. Gordins dedicated herself to daycare so that she could contently watch over her grandson and other babies from the apartment complex, while Julia once again began teaching piano lessons; the money they earned allowed them to hire a first-rate housekeeper and cook as well as to provide the mother and daughter with greater financial freedom and personal happiness. Gilman's story made clear her belief that allowing household labor to specialize, as if the home were a modern business, would free women of all ages from the mental and physical burden of fulfilling traditional domestic duties for which they were ill suited. Just as important, granting more freedom in domestic responsibility would also give women the opportunity to avoid idleness, to cultivate personal interests, to develop useful skills, and ultimately to help create stronger, more tightly-knit communities—all themes she addressed more fully in her landmark *Women and Economics* (1898).[58]

One of Gilman's most succinct products linking gender roles to neurasthenia was her 1916 essay "The 'Nervous Breakdown' of Women," wherein she took issue with the claim of physicians such as Mitchell that women became nervous wrecks because they spent too much energy pursuing "outside interests" rather than following "natural domestic ones." Students and farmer's wives alike were prone to neurasthenic breakdowns, she argued, thus it was erroneous to blame the condition simply on intellectual activity. Healthy nerves came from the smooth interaction between the "body" and the "spirit"; problems arose when social expectations forced women to do domestic jobs for which they were not intellectually or spiritually suited. The result, she concluded, was a population of American women plagued by neurasthenia.[59] Gilman essentially turned convention on its ear as she located the cause for women's unhappiness and discomfort *inside* the domestic sphere rather than *outside*. Paralleling in many ways Mason's reprimand of Mitchell for disparaging women physicians, Gilman explained how healthy women needed greater leeway in determining what jobs, domestic or otherwise, best suited their physical and intellectual abilities. With talented women free to dedicate their efforts to national causes, Gilman believed America would progress far beyond other nations socially, economically, and culturally.[60]

The idealism of Homes and Beecher—that domesticity ultimately benefitted women—foundered on the reality that rigid female gender roles could be harmful to the mental and physical well-being of women. The American medical profession was not entirely ignorant of this. In 1886 (the same year Gilman suffered from neurasthenia following the birth of her daughter), Dr. Grace Peckham presented a paper in front of the reform-minded American Social Science Association stressing the need for women to have outlets for intellectual and creative endeavors. "It is more often lack of mental culture which reacts upon the physical condition of women," she explained to her mostly male colleagues; "My hope of relief for those who are suffering from extreme nervousness is based upon the amount of interest which can be aroused for some intellectual pursuit." Something needed to be done, she argued, to relieve women of their "never-ending routine of petty duties."[61] Mitchell mostly agreed with Peckham, as he supported Mason's and Wister's activities outside the home and in his writings stressed the need for women to have diversionary interests. Gilman's experience with Mitchell demonstrated, however, that the doctor did not apply this principle to all his patients evenly.

Perhaps the most practical understanding of the need for women to branch out from their conventional household roles came from yet another neurasthenic patient of Mitchell's: Jane Addams, the founder of the American settlement house movement. In an 1893 essay titled "The Subjective Necessity for Social Settlements," Addams explained how marriage too often gave a woman a "sense of uselessness" that removed "something vital out of her life to which she is entitled." Addams envisioned settlement houses as opportunities for young women to pursue active lives, relationships, and happiness outside of marriage, while also helping relieve the burden of poverty in American cities. By 1910, the idea that domesticity represented a genuine health threat had gained currency, as *Harper's Bazaar* reported on unfortunate housewives who "fall into a state of depression, develop nerves, lose the taste of life, [and] sometimes become seriously ill."[62] Depression, anxiety, pain—these were all neurasthenic symptoms experienced one time or another by Mason, Wister, and Gilman, whose personal struggle with the disease led them to realize that for women to live healthy, happy, and comfortable lives, gender roles needed to be expanded to allow them greater opportunity to follow their interests and talents.

Neurasthenia was a gendered affair, and one's sex had a profound impact on how a neurasthenic reflected on the illness. Perhaps due to their dominant social position, men were less willing than women to fault convention for their illness and had a tendency to interpret their neurasthenia as the result of weak wills rather than of broken gender roles. For men, neurasthenia often came with shame over a perceived lack of manliness that drew into question their ability to be productive, to support their families, and to control their emotions, thoughts, and sexuality. This warranted personal adjustment, such as engaging in masculine activity or reevaluating dedication to work and family (in addition to the typical electrotherapy and drug treatments). Women, who by tradition enjoyed fewer rights and privileges, were more likely to attribute their neurasthenia to flawed gendered roles and consequently used their health issues to challenge social convention in the hopes of securing women greater opportunity to pursue a life outside the restraints of domesticity. Establishing their role as public caretakers of a national culture, asserting their need for relaxation away from the family, and arguing for more flexibility in working outside the home were not only issues of women's rights, but also issues of personal health.

On a larger level, the experiences of Dreiser, the author of "Autobiography of a Neurasthenic," Mason, Wister, and Gilman were representative of broader social movements taking place in turn-of-the-century America. Dreiser's experience at Muldoon's Farm, for instance, was representative of the "physical culture" movement that was gaining ground in the nation at the time and that encouraged people to look to exercise and diet as keys to happier, healthier lives. "Autobiography of a Neurasthenic" echoed the message that advocates of companionate marriage had been making for decades: that the healthiest families are those in which the husband and wife work together as supportive parents. Mason's call for women to be socially active and strengthen the national culture paralleled the women's club movement, which Jane C. Croly and Julia Ward Howe helped found as a way of allowing women to reach their intellectual and cultural potential. Wister's reliance on resorts to recuperate from draining housework spoke to a growing tradition that would blossom in the twentieth century as Americans developed a taste for vacations. Gilman's call to restructure domestic work to allow women more freedom followed in the footsteps of America's many "Bellamy Societies" influenced by Edward Bellamy's best-seller *Looking Backwards* (1888), which featured a utopian future in which each man and woman could work at jobs for which they were perfectly adapted.[63]

Neurasthenia created situations that encouraged people to reevaluate society and advocate changes in the hope of avoiding the chronic illness. As promoters and advertisers discovered, a person did not have to be afflicted with the condition to be influenced by it; the threat alone of the disease proved enough to convince Americans to modify their daily habits to try to counteract the enervating effects of modern life that might lead to it. Consequently, by the end of the nineteenth century, Americans were in the process of switching their attention from how to *treat* neurasthenia to how to *prevent* it altogether. This attempt to be proactive in the fight against neurasthenia fed the development of modern therapeutic lifestyles built on the ideas of health, happiness, and comfort.

Chapter 5

Lifestyle and Managing the Healthy Balance

In his light-hearted book *Confession of a Neurasthenic* (1908), Dr. William Taylor Marrs detailed the life of a genteel man dedicated to the pursuit of health. Spoiled as a child and consequently impatient and easily bored as an adult, the fictional narrator constantly jumped from one career path and fad to the next, hoping to find contentment. "Indecision marked my life and character and I had no confidence in myself," he admitted.[1] By describing his condition, the narrator hoped to demonstrate that he was in fact a tragically ill man in need of sympathy, not a shiftless slouch deserving of scorn. His "misdirected" mind wandered toward morbid fears and hypochondrias if left unoccupied, thus making his life a long, often absurd attempt to find health by going through one therapeutic lifestyle change after another. He tried his hand at being a farmer, a journalist, an athlete, a vegetarian, a cowboy, a doctor, a foundry laborer, a public speaker, a follower of New Thought, a correspondence school administrator, and finally an author—which is where the book abruptly ended, when the narrator reported that he had at last lost interest in finishing his story.

Marrs's book is a comment on how neurasthenia prompted people to search for new ways of living to improve their quality of life. "Lifestyle" is an anachronistic term that Marrs himself did not use, but it is helpful to describe how people began engaging in activities that were not immediately profitable (they tended to cost money rather than to make it) but were therapeutic and helped make life bearable, if not rewarding.[2] To an extent, having the freedom to modify one's lifestyle emerged from the late nineteenth century as a liberal hallmark of America's middle class: education was becoming more accessible to boys, girls, men, and women; sports leagues and athletics became wide-spread;

railroads allowed inexpensive travel in and out of cities; and an expanding, yet rocky, economy afforded more money to spend on activities of choice. There were, of course, serious limitations on who could participate in these new developments, with racial prejudice and poverty being important barriers. Another was America's tradition of hard work and distaste for malingering—a tradition identified by German sociologist Max Weber in 1904 as part of the "Protestant work ethic"—that discouraged people from living lives that might be considered too leisurely.[3]

Neurasthenia, however, helped Americans ignore the stigma of malingering by making lifestyle changes a medical imperative rather than a whimsical desire to avoid work. The illness caused people to realize that modern facets of life—city dwelling, sedentary lives, office jobs, competitive business practices, intense education, to name a few—needed to be balanced with therapeutic activities. The anxiety of studying for final exams could be lifted with a rigorous afternoon of playing football, for instance, or a week of tiring social engagements could be balanced with a weekend bike ride. Although some of these lifestyle changes retained the elements of rest that S. Weir Mitchell had stressed for neurasthenics since the early 1870s, generally these new therapeutic lifestyles became more active as the turn of the century approached. This shift toward activity began gaining momentum in the 1880s in American schools, where compulsory attendance laws combined with competitive curricula to make reformers and parents fear that heavy-handed academics would stifle natural childhood development and produce generations of weakling children suffering from overwork, worry, and neurasthenia. The healthy solution was the development of physical education classes as a counterweight. Indeed, by late century a physical culture movement had developed that promised to compensate for the neurasthenia-inducing effects of modern society. Concern over neurasthenia also helped justify the late-century resurgence in anti-modern lifestyles, such as delving into handicrafts and spending holidays "getting back to nature," far removed from enervating city life. There was no way to push back time and return to a neurasthenia-free, premodern society, but Americans did what they could to manage the draining anxiety of modern life in the hope of achieving health, happiness, and comfort.

Neurasthenia, Public Education, and Athletics

One of the most fundamental changes happening in late-nineteenth-century America was the growth of public education. The nation had a long tradition of public schooling tracing back to New England Puritan settlements, but during the second half of the nineteenth century the quantity of students, money, and

attention dedicated to public education swelled, thanks to compulsory attendance laws aimed at children from eight to fourteen years old. Massachusetts
was the first to issue such a law in 1852, and by 1918, when Mississippi passed
legislation, every state had an equivalent law.[4] How the expanding school systems would develop was not altogether clear to educators at the time, as an
educational initiative as ambitious as this had never been attempted. Difficult
questions loomed, including the content of school curricula, the viability of
coeducation, the role of homework, and whether classrooms should seek the
successes—and anxieties—of a competitive work environment. Neurasthenia
played the role of educational boogeyman and generated a heated debate among
parents, educators, and physicians that result in an educational strategy of
balancing rigorous academics with exercise, school design, and teacher training.

According to many late-century physicians, just as adult nerves were
threatened by pressure and responsibility, so too were children's nerves threatened by mandatory education. This is not to imply that physicians thought
universal education was a bad thing. On the contrary, the expansion of public
education was widely seen as a good thing by physicians; concern was over
finding the *healthiest* form of education. To this end, Mitchell dedicated a substantial portion of *Wear and Tear* to the issue of childhood education and strong
nerves, and the Massachusetts Emergency and Hygiene Association gave a
series of lectures in 1884 for the state's schoolteachers on the topic "School
Hygiene." In these lectures, association vice-president Dr. Frank Wells listed
nervous diseases as one of the top five threats to public schoolchildren, the other
four being epidemic diseases, eyestrain, poor drainage in school buildings, and
poor heating and ventilation. Physicians and school reformers even looked to
their colleagues across the Atlantic, such as British physician James Crichton-
Browne and his studies on "over-pressure in schools," and to the innovative
educational theories by Johann Heinrich Pestalozzi and Friedrich Froebel coming out of Central Europe. In the opinion of many, there was an inescapable
connection between education and health, and if school systems were going to
take responsibility for the former, they also had to take responsibility for the
latter. "A sound nervous system is undoubtedly a most important factor . . . [in]
an individual's . . . education," Dr. Charles Mills pointed out to schoolteachers
and medical colleagues. This relationship between nerves and education was
reciprocal, Mills insisted, as "a good education will do more than anything else
to develop and strengthen the nervous system."[5]

Late-nineteenth-century physicians and educators cited a handful of reasons why schools threatened the health of students. One was overwork. Given the
general belief that children required vital energy to fuel mental and physical

growth, reformers were concerned that competitive students and those eager to please their parents or teachers would overexert themselves with school work, thereby draining their bodies of energy and stunting their intellectual and physical growth. "Overwork is especially dangerous," Dr. Horatio Wood warned parents and teachers in 1882, because it allowed the "terrible possibility of diverting energy which should be spent in development . . . thereby dwarfing the brain itself." It was during this time that many schools launched more rigorous curricula by expanding the scope of arithmetic, science, and government lessons, consequently fueling concerns that children's nervous systems could not balance all this academic, intellectual, and physical growth. A rather prickly situation developed for educators who were supposed to get students to think—but not too much. Boston City Hospital's Dr. Charles Follen Folsom, for instance, cautioned teachers that "excitable, precocious children" were more likely to fall victim to nervous disorders because they risked being "overstimulated." "The fact is too often overlooked," he warned, "that intellectual brightness in children may be only a symptom of illness."[6] Mediocrity evidently had its benefits.

In addition to risking overburdening children with brainwork, educational reformers feared, schools might become "over-pressured" environments that weakened children's minds with anxiety. Examinations, exhibitions, and school performances alarmed some physicians and teachers, who believed that these activities did more to sap than to fortify students' confidence and mental stability. "If we could do without examinations altogether," Mitchell lectured an audience of Philadelphia schoolteachers, "it would be hygienically a distinct gain." Incentives such as prizes, class rankings, and promotion to the next grade level ratcheted up the pressure, causing many students to develop what Mitchell characterized as "morbid fears" that, he said, drained them of energy and left them languishing with nervous afflictions. According to the Massachusetts Board of Education, part of this problem was due to large classroom sizes (forty or more students) that encouraged arbitrary standards, forced unfair comparisons among students of differing abilities, and prevented lessons from being tailored to individual "capacity and needs." Fred Atkinson, the principal of the Springfield, Massachusetts, high school, believed in the necessity of keeping exams as a labor-saving device for teachers, but advocated the elimination of grades and a transition to a simple "pass/not pass" system to reduce student anxiety.[7]

The alarms raised by physicians such as Mitchell, Folsom, Wells, and Wood resonated with Americans. An editorial in *Health Magazine* called public education a "menace to the future health of the community" by reportedly driving students to suicide by subjecting them to the "same fierce competition that pervades the commercial world." Principal Atkinson, in an 1897 article published in the *School Review*, observed that "in the public mind" overexertion and overanxiety were the "greatest" dangers to the health of schoolchildren. During his tenure as principal, Atkinson had to deal with numerous parental complaints that the anxiety of high school hurt their children. Some examples: "I should think the high-school teachers were trying to kill my boy"; "If I wanted to ruin my daughter's health, I would send her to the high school"; "My daughter was graduated from the high school with honors, but I had to have her rest a year before allowing her to go to college." Writer and poet Bertha E. Bush reported in the *Christian Advocate* that "many a tirade against the modern school-system" arose from the prevalent "hackneyed assertion" that schooling harmed girls' ability to develop into healthy women.[8]

Coeducation created a particularly difficult situation for educators, as many considered girls more susceptible to overwork and pressure than boys. Harvard professor Edward Clarke questioned the wisdom of coeducation in his widely read 1873 study *Sex in Education; or, A Fair Chance for the Girls*, which argued that it was patently unfair to expect girls to be able to compete with boys in school. To put boys and girls in the same classes supposedly strained young girls' capacities and undermined their ability to develop into healthy wives and mothers. Far wiser, Clarke argued, would be to educate girls separately from boys, so that they could develop at their own natural pace. In tacit agreement, Wells argued that grades provoked "nervous emotions, such as fear of failure [and] over-excitation at success" among girls "to a much greater degree than with boys." Mitchell disagreed with Clarke and Wells on this, believing boys and girls had similar capacities to learn and deal with the pressures of schools, with girls' greater maturity even giving them a slight advantage. However, once girls entered adolescence and began to develop sexually, Mitchell believed, they needed to avoid the competitive demands of education until after puberty, lest they permanently weaken themselves and impair their ability to raise healthy children. This danger not only threatened young women on an individual basis, but, according to Mitchell, also threatened the entire nation by (supposedly) lowering birth rates and increasing the number of sickly children.[9]

Faced with the potential threats of dwarfed brains, neurasthenic breakdowns, and infertility among students, educators sought to enact changes to make schools safer for the students and their delicate nervous systems. Changes had to be adopted cautiously because reformers feared that simply making classes easier and less competitive might be counterproductive. Folsom insisted that teachers needed to help students "meet and conquer" obstacles rather than simply "evade" them; in this way, children would be better prepared to deal with adversity and anxiety during adulthood. He warned that sometimes teachers catered too readily to students' claims of overexertion, especially the claims made by girls, thereby inadvertently encouraging children to become lazy, unambitious, and chronic invalids—not the sort of people poised to live successful lives.[10] The challenge for reformers was to develop an educational system that allowed for enough competition and difficulty to cultivate resilience and strong character among the students, while also protecting their vulnerable nervous systems and vital energy. Children were to be kept healthy but not coddled.

Reformers concerned with neurasthenia did not lower academic expectations so much as they sought to help students meet those expectations by strengthening young nervous systems. To this end, physical education and exercise became imperative. Experts at the time believed that developing students' physiques—strength, agility, lung capacity, and pulse—was the best way to increase their capacity to produce and store the vital energy necessary to succeed in school. Powerful bodies, the logic went, could better sustain powerful minds. This was not an entirely new idea, as gymnastic advocates such as Dioclesian "Dio" Lewis (1823–1886) had been vehemently campaigning for physical education since the 1860s, but the threat of neurasthenia brought new urgency to the calls. Mitchell urged schools to make ten minutes of every hour a time of recess in which young students had to leave the classroom and be active, if not in natural play then at least in the form of coordinated gymnastics. Folsom recommended that American schools look to Germany and that nation's decision to incorporate physical education into the curriculum as fully as it did math and geography. "This is a thousand times better," he argued in front of the Massachusetts Teacher's Association, "than all the rest cures and mind cures" that doctors typically recommended to neurasthenics.[11]

In addition to keeping students physically fit, school reformers aimed to fortify young nervous systems by improving classroom ventilation and children's diets. Stuffy, poorly circulated air, all too common in urban schools, was thought to lack the vital nutrients found in fresh air. At the behest of reformers, many districts began renovating schools to improve air circulation, a movement that Charles Mills, the president of the American Neurological Association, thought in 1886 was going in the right direction. Similarly, common sense dictated that what students ate and drank had a direct bearing on their generation of vital energy. Folsom contended that from either poverty or neglect, many students arrived in school not having had a proper breakfast or carrying a nutritious lunch. He urged—and districts began to listen—that schools universally sell milk to children during breaks, a side business that janitors at the time typically ran to make extra money. By 1900, new elementary schools began to follow a more or less standard layout that incorporated centralized ventilation and set aside substantial space for lunchrooms, playrooms, playgrounds or gymnasiums, and showers. Concerned educators and physicians also founded the International Congress of School Hygiene, which discussed topics such as the "hygiene of school building" when they met in London in 1907 and in Buffalo, New York, in 1913.[12]

Finally, teachers and parents assumed the additional responsibility of keeping a closer eye on the health of their students and children. Although teachers had long been on the lookout for contagious diseases, by the 1880s nervous diseases increasingly became part of their agendas. Administrators consulted with neurologists to give in-service training on how to identify the behavioral and emotional signs of nervous diseases in children; such training occurred at the 1884 annual meeting of the Massachusetts Teachers' Association.[13] Articles written in educational journals by administrators such as Atkinson reminded teachers of the need to keep a close watch over "special individuals," especially "the sensitively conscientious girl." Popular health manuals, such as Horatio Wood's *Brain-Work and Overwork* (1882), sprang up as well, seeking to "diffuse as widely and cheaply as possible" information on the prevention and cure of nervous illness to help people "take care of themselves, their children, [and] pupils."[14] Cognizant of the threat posed by neurasthenia, the educational community and concerned parents began taking issues of health, especially nervous health, more seriously.

Public concern over schooling and neurasthenia revealed deep-seated racial assumptions within America's turn-of-the-century education system. Fears that competitive education might lead to neurasthenic children were limited almost entirely to white communities because, with few exceptions, the educational experience of black students was not so academically rigorous as that of middle-class white students. Part of the reason for this arose from the belief that black Americans' proper social and economic roles were as laborers, not as educated professionals. Endorsed by leaders such as Booker T. Washington in his 1895 "Atlanta Compromise," America's dominant educational policy for blacks stressed the need for industrial and vocational training rather than for the academic training white students more often received. Although part of the focus on vocational training came from black Americans' rural identity (an estimated 73 percent lived in agrarian areas in 1916), much of it also came from persistent racist expectations. Echoing sensibilities that would have supported slavery a generation before, some observers contended that it was the national duty of blacks to provide America with a reliable and steady labor force. "If our

civilization is to continue," wrote Robert Lewis Dabney of Virginia's Union
Theological Seminary, "there must be, at the bottom of the social fabric, a class
who must work and not read." Dabney used the language of neurasthenia to justify his position: "The people [i.e., blacks] who are addicted to manual labor are
never going to be students. . . . The brain which is taxed to supply the nervous
energy for a day of manual labor, will have none left for literary pursuits."[15]
Simply put, the purpose of the American educational system was to teach
blacks to be farmers, carpenters, and bricklayers—manual careers many thought
little affected by neurasthenia—rather than neurasthenia-prone doctors, lawyers,
or bankers.

Another reason why black students were left out of the discussion surrounding neurasthenia was their reputation for not taking school as strenu-
ously, and thus as nervously, as white students. Sociologist W. E. B. Du Bois
explained black apathy toward schools as the natural product of the segregated
system that limited students to futures as manual laborers rather than give them
the opportunity to become professionals. "There has risen up a policy of harsh
repression and gentle discouragement toward you, me and the children we
teach," Du Bois explained in a 1906 speech to black educators at Virginia's
Hampton Institute, a flagship school for Booker T. Washington's industrial education movement. Du Bois, a staunch opponent of Washington's educational
philosophy, called vocational training "educational heresy" because it encouraged young blacks "not to hitch their wagons to a star, but to a mule," thus
deemphasizing intellectual pursuits and academic competition, those activities
that supposedly sparked neurasthenia among white students.[16]

By 1916 even the federal government recognized the demoralized state of
the nation's black elementary and secondary schools, which received on average only a quarter of the funds per student received by white schools. A
national Bureau of Education study concluded that something needed to be done
to "arouse the colored people" to better "appreciate" the value of education.
For elementary schools, this meant additional funding. For secondary schools,
the study ironically concluded that curricula needed to focus on "simplicity"
and even more manual training because "the Negro's highly emotional nature
requires for balance as much as possible of the concrete and definite."[17] By
characterizing blacks as "highly emotional," the Bureau of Education reinforced the perception that blacks were a savage, primitive race that operated by
emotional instinct rather than intelligent rationality (and consequently were
presumably not at risk of developing neurasthenia).

What did the national discussion over education and neurasthenia mean for
American children growing up during the late nineteenth and early twentieth

centuries? For black children, the assumption was that they would use their hands and prepare for life as laborers, an experience that encouraged them to become just the sort of adults that neurasthenia pioneer George M. Beard estimated were too brutish to be neurasthenic. For white children, the threat of neurasthenia in the classroom stood as an informal badge of racial distinction and evidence of the students' intellectual, competitive natures, but it also raised the issue of whether the educational system was pushing them too hard and subjecting them to the same enervating demands that adults experienced in the modern competitive world. What is more, although there were some calls to reduce the academic load placed on these children, school reformers generally accepted academic competition as a beneficial rehearsal for adulthood, and instead chose to redirect reforms toward strengthening children's nervous systems through exercise, school design, and teacher awareness. "If we can develop and train a race of men and women possessing good digestion, a tough muscular system and sound health; a steady, firm nervous system which can bear the stress and strain, and meet the emergencies of life," Amherst's John Tyler wrote in the *School Review*, "we may well be proud of our work."[18]

Physical Culture and the Strenuous Life

Physical education was emblematic of a larger physical culture movement taking place in America. The decades following the Civil War witnessed an explosion of sports teams and a fetishistic fascination with exercise and bodily health. A fundamental reason for this late-century fascination with athletics was a persistent fear that urban civilization had transformed Americans into a degenerate race of weaklings, of which neurasthenia was an indication. Sports were seen as a way of strengthening people's vital spirits and physical bodies while also teaching the Victorian virtues of restraint and order. What is more, for a population that increasingly lived in cities and worked indoors, athletics served as a chance to get outside, breathe fresh air, and benefit from the restorative powers of nature.[19]

Interest in organized sports grew spectacularly during the late nineteenth century, prompting critics to wonder if the pendulum between academics and athletics had swung too far and sports were causing more harm than good. The National Association of Base Ball Players established itself in 1867, followed by the Rowing Association of America (1871), the National Bowling League (1875), and the National Association of Amateur Athletes of America (1879). American colleges in particular felt the presence of sports teams, as East Coast schools such as Harvard, Yale, Rutgers, Columbia, and Pennsylvania developed vibrant student-led clubs for rowing, football, baseball, and track and field throughout the 1870s and 1880s. Student enthusiasm for their teams became so fervent that some observers feared that sports threatened to eclipse academics on American campuses. Princeton president James McCosh argued as early as 1883 that collegiate sports had become counterproductive and that student discussion of games and athletes had replaced erudite talk of science, philosophy, and literature. Harvard president Charles Eliot also battled to control the violent and obsessive nature of collegiate sports, particularly football. Mitchell, ever ready to give his opinion on social matters, weighed in on the issue during a 1906 address to University of Pennsylvania alumni: "We old fellows get a little impatient about the absorbing interest the college man has in bodily contests, and his general indifference to the triumph of the mental athlete."[20] In the push to increase athletics to allow more intellectual activity, balance was not always kept and sometimes brawn overshadowed brain.

While collegiate sports were gaining a notorious reputation, a less bellicose athletic spirit was spreading through American cities with the "muscular Christianity" movement. From its beginnings in Britain as a midcentury literary movement, muscular Christianity grew among Americans in response to the fear that they had become an overcivilized, enervated nation where men had lost their manly spirit. American advocates such as minister Josiah Strong, Theodore Roosevelt, and psychologist G. Stanley Hall sought to combine athleticism and religious faith not only to invigorate a population wracked by nervous illness, but also to strengthen the nation around the same Anglo-Saxon population that Beard had identified with neurasthenia. The Young Men's Christian Association (YMCA) spearheaded the movement by providing gymnasiums, swimming pools, and sporting opportunities to urbanites, even designing new indoor games such as basketball (1891) and volleyball (1896) so that those in cities could enjoy the vitalizing influence of team sports all year long. Luther H. Gulick, described by one historian as "the greatest of YMCA philosophers," designed the organization's official seal (an inverted red triangle) to symbolize the symmetric relationship among body, mind, and spirit—three interrelated elements that neurasthenics so often found in disarray.[21]

By no means were late-century athletics exclusively a manly hobby, as women at the time also had reasons for incorporating exercise into their lifestyles. *Godey's Magazine*, that epitome of American domestic sensibility, claimed that "highly strained" modern lifestyles put American women at heightened risk for nervous prostration and its side effects, including premature aging and unattractive lethargy. "Paint, powder and stimulants," the magazine stated, "would not be needed by women if they took regular daily exercise out-of-doors, in a gymnasium, or even at home with light dumb bells, pulley weights or free hand movements." For those who feared exercise might be a tad manly, *Godey's* stressed its feminine aspects by suggesting that "men desire health, strength and grace in a woman just as much as a pretty face." Illustrator Charles Dana Gibson capitalized on this connection between exercise and womanly beauty in his many "Gibson Girl" illustrations; engaged in sports such as golfing and swimming, the independent Gibson Girl stood in stark contrast to the neurasthenic invalid, wielding a seductive power that sprang from her glowing health.[22]

Exercise meant more to women than simply staying healthy and attractive; advocates argued that it also fortified their nervous energy so that they could take a more active role in American society. At its 1894 annual meeting, members of the New York branch of Sorosis (one of the first and most influential clubs dedicated to the professional, intellectual, and social advancement of women) met to listen to music and discuss the topic of nervousness among modern women. Addressing the audience, Dr. Madana Fuller De Hart, an advocate for young women's educational and health needs, claimed that part of the cause of neurasthenia lay with inequalities within the educational system that

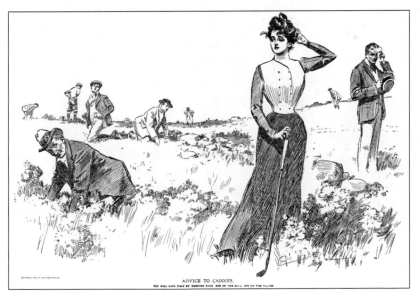

Figure 12   Charles Dana Gibson, *Advice to Caddies: You Will Save Time by Keeping Your Eye on the Ball*, 1900. "Gibson Girl" images such as this helped normalize the idea that women who engaged in outdoor sport and exercise could be models of healthy feminine beauty.

From *The Gibson Book: A Collection of the Published Works of Charles Dana Gibson* [New York: C. Scribner's Sons, 1906].

assigned girls to learn poetry while boys learned math and science, thereby causing "abnormal development" of women's emotions at the expense of their rationality. Educational reforms needed to take place to correct this problem, but in the meantime, De Hart told her audience, the "physical culture that is now the fashion will prove the foundation of a lasting reform. . . . Let us not forget that in our climate we need work to preserve health and soul and body. With that we need plenty of sleep, regular hours, sunlight, fresh air and exercise." Charlotte Perkins Gilman, too, had recognized the therapeutic value of outdoor activities in recovering from neurasthenia: "Kind and congenial friends, pleasant society, amusement, out-door sports, the blessed mountains . . . with such surroundings I recovered so fast."[23] By 1900 exercise had become a hallmark of America's vital, energetic "New Woman" and distinguished her from the domestic, neurasthenic women of previous generations.

Bicycles were the darling of this late nineteenth-century athletic craze and quickly became a favorite form of exercise among women as well as men. In 1885 Englishman John Kemp Starley transformed the bicycle from the rickety, high-wheeled "penny-farthing" to the rear-wheel-drive, chain-driven bike known as the Rover Safety Bicycle. In 1888 Scotsman John Dunlop developed the pneumatic tire, which reduced riding's jarring bumpiness, and in 1895 a German immigrant to the United States, Ignaz Schwinn, established a bicycle factory in Chicago that fitted bike seats with springs to make the ride even more smooth. Also at this time, Henry Clyde wrote the bicycle handbook *Pleasure-Cycling* (1895) and declared that the amusement was on the verge of becoming America's "national sport," a claim that the *New York Observer and Chronicle* took a step further when it asked the question "Will all the world ride the bicycle?" The newspaper estimated that, in 1896, New York City alone had 200,000 bike riders, while the United States as a whole had approximately 4 million riders— nearly 6 percent of the nation's total population. With numbers like this, biking had displaced horseback riding as America's preferred mode of personal transportation, according to the paper. Women in particular were recognized for their dedication: "To them the wheel has brought a new freedom, emancipation from the monotony of household routine and from convention of dress, the reason no doubt that they enjoy it even more than the men."[24] The bike was a symbol of therapeutic exercise not only of the physical body, but of personal freedom as well.

When it came to combating neurasthenia, bicycles represented a healthy opportunity to replenish spent nerves and calm troublesome thoughts. "Dullness, lassitude, headache, fly away on the breeze which your own motion creates," Clyde explained to readers in *Pleasure-Cycling*. "Over-wrought and weary"

businessmen could rely on bicycling to improve their strength, soothe digestion, and make "nerves less importunate." "The bicycle has been the greatest of
blessings to my husband," a wife of a bike enthusiast informed Clyde; "He has
always seemed fairly well, but always nervous, and at times afflicted with the
worst attacks of 'the blues.' They never visit him now in the wheeling season."
Bicycle advertisers, who helped propel America's biking phenomenon of
the 1890s, also alluded to the sport's ability to pacify a distraught mind. "A
DISORDERED BRAIN evolves strange fancies," announced an ad for Keating Wheel
Company, while "A WELL ORDERED BRAIN, with the aid of science, evolved the
19 lb KEATING." Speaking at the thirty-fourth commencement of the Eclectic

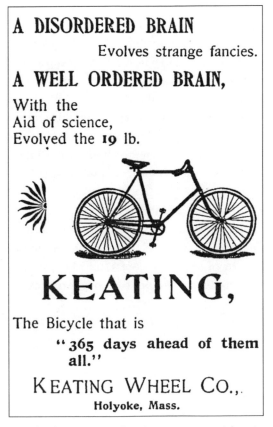

A DISORDERED BRAIN

Evolves strange fancies.

A WELL ORDERED BRAIN,

With the
Aid of science,
Evolved the **19** lb.

KEATING,

The Bicycle that is
    " **365** days ahead of them
    all.''

K EATING W HEEL C O.,.
Holyoke, Mass.

Figure 13   Keating Wheel Company advertisement, 1895. Advertisers and promoters
marketed bicycles as enjoyable exercise for women and men that invigorated the body
and strengthened the nervous system and mind. Bicycling riding was one of many
turn-of-the-century health habits that Americans developed to fortify themselves against
neurasthenia.

From *Current Literature* 17 [June 1895]: 13.

Medical College of New York, which graduated five women and nine men, the Rev. Dr. D. Asa Blackburn expressed some tongue-in-cheek concern that bicycling was siphoning off the finest medical school talent: "If the new woman wants to find an outlet for her surplus energy, vim, and brain force, here is the place, and not upon the bicycle."[25] By the turn of the century, biking was synonymous with the lifestyles of young, healthy, and ambitious individuals full of vital nervous energy and determined to improve their lives.

America's obsession with physical culture culminated in the rise of Theodore Roosevelt as a national icon. In an 1899 address before the Hamilton Club in Chicago, Roosevelt contended that if the United States were to take its place as a leader among nations, citizens needed to follow the strenuous life. "In the last analysis," Roosevelt lectured his audience, "a healthy state can exist only when the men and women who make it up lead clean, vigorous, healthy lives." He tried to do the same himself. The year 1884 was a difficult one for him, as both his mother and wife died—hours apart, on Valentine's Day. The sudden loss left him emotionally devastated and also concerned that he might inherit the cancer and neurasthenia that had plagued others in his family. Needing to distance himself from personal calamity and rejuvenate himself, he moved to the Dakota Territory where he operated a cattle ranch, served as a law officer, and indeed lived a "strenuous life." "I have never been in better health," he wrote his older sister Anna; "I am in the saddle all day long either taking part in the round up of cattle, or else hunting antelope." When he returned to East Coast politics in 1886, the man previously known as a young dandy with a shrill voice had reinvented himself as a rugged cowboy of boundless energy capable of tackling problems around the nation and the globe. An amateur boxer, fan of collegiate sports, and big-game hunter, Roosevelt personified the turn-of-the-century drive among Americans to be people of action.[26]

Riding on the coattails of Roosevelt's celebrity, the active life became America's fashionable turn-of-the-century answer to neurasthenia. According to a 1905 *New York Times* article, "The Strenuous Side of Social Life at Our National Capital," Washington wives in the Roosevelt Administration were falling prey to demanding, hectic schedules. "Nervous prostration is the spectre which haunts nearly all women who have to endure the grinding fatigue of a Washington official season," the *Times* reported. According to the article, the strains of hosting dinners and entertaining political dignitaries had reduced three cabinet wives and a daughter to near-invalidism, prompting political women throughout Washington to modify their lifestyles to avoid neurasthenia. For instance, Edith Roosevelt (the president's second wife), "like her distinguished husband, finds a panacea for all ills in open-air exercise." Unlike the president, she did not hunt big game or rope cattle—instead, she went on "shopping expeditions." "Mrs. Roosevelt does not believe in aimless walking, even for exercise," the *Times* explained. Shopping allowed her the opportunity of hours of walking as well as the chance to keep her mind "intelligently employed" thinking of what gifts to buy for her friends and family. Helen Taft, a "fragile-looking woman" and wife of Secretary of War William Howard Taft, engaged in a more traditional sport, rowing eight to ten miles a day with her sixteen-year-old son. Clara Root, a "delicate woman" and wife of Secretary of State Elihu Root, took to studying French and German to steady her "shattered nerves," while her daughter, Edith Root, delighted in cross-country running and "rough-and-ready" horseback riding with Roosevelt when the president desired a "genial companion." Finally, the *Times* featured the habits of Lillie Knox, wife of former Attorney General Philander Knox, who had "conquered her nerves" by spending winters in Florida, where she "luxuriated in the land of the alligators," before assuming the strenuous job of managing a Pennsylvania dairy farm. Between supervising the milking, doing the churning herself, and studying the latest scientific works on agriculture, Knox "forgot all about headaches, sleepless nights, or the inclination to start at imaginary noises or to weep for nothing at all."[27] By shopping, rowing, and running a farm, the women of Washington demonstrated to their nation that there were many ways to remain active and beat the neurasthenia blues.

When Secretary of State Root, whose wife studied languages and whose daughter galloped with the president, collapsed from neurasthenia in 1907, there was no talk of rest cure. If he was to recover, it would be via the strenuous life. The official word from the White House was that Secretary Root had been long suffering from nervous exhaustion caused by overwork and his meticulous application to detail. The unofficial story from Wall Street insiders was that Roosevelt's "trust busting" had placed an unbearable strain on Root, who had close friends in corporate America and whose influence within the administration was being supplanted by other cabinet members such as Secretary of War Taft and Secretary of Treasury George Cortelyou. Regardless of the exact reasons for Root's neurasthenia, newspapers reported that Roosevelt personally took him to Muldoon's Farm in White Plains, New York—the same place Theodore Dreiser went to recover from his neurasthenia—to make sure Root received the most strenuous cure possible. William Muldoon described Root's initial condition to reporters as "very weak and feeble," saying, "He was suffering from mental exhaustion, his nervous energy was worn out, and his brain was tired. He was anxious about matters that should not have worried him. When he went to bed his mind was worried about things that did not exist."[28] Root was spent, and needed to be recharged to carry on the nation's work.

If reports are to be trusted, in five weeks Muldoon worked Root back into shape with a rigorous regime befitting an Olympic athlete. The sixty-two-year-old Root engaged in a daily schedule "as strenuous as the Administration of which he is part," including twenty miles of horseback riding, three to five miles of walking, and a couple of hours of boxing. It is unclear whether Root did the morning milking, a typical task for patients on the farm. Muldoon proudly announced to the press that, under his tutelage, Root was quickly improving and gaining one pound a day. "If the president calls a meeting of the Cabinet," Muldoon mused to reporters, "Mr. Root will be, with the exception of the president only, about the strongest man around the table, not even barring the marvelously vigorous Secretary of War." (The secretary of war was future president William Howard Taft, who, at six feet and 340 pounds, was marvelously vigorous indeed!) The results clearly impressed Roosevelt, who a few months later also sent the chief of the army general staff, Brig. Gen. James Franklin Bell, to Muldoon's to recover from a neurasthenic breakdown (reportedly also caused by overwork and worry).[29] Roosevelt did not try to hide the neurasthenia within his administration; to the contrary, he used it as evidence that he ran a vigorous, dedicated government—from the Washington wives to the cabinet members— who were willing to literally work themselves sick for the American people.

In New Jersey, a "Muldoon's for women" allowed "school teachers, settlement workers, and business women" of all ages to "cure their shattered nerves" through exercise. Every morning, patients worked on "pumping," a breathing technique that relied on abdominal muscles, followed by "the scissors," lying full-length on one side and moving the legs as if they were shears, and various gymnastics, such as somersaults and hand stands. These activities reportedly brought about remarkable results, including one legendary instance in which a patient who had been "for many years an invalid" celebrated her renewed health by standing on her head on the back of a horse doing circles in a riding ring. Afternoons were dedicated to such athletic activities as rowing, swimming, and bareback "rough riding" that allowed women to exercise outdoors and forget their troubles. The weakest patients could make do by taking nature walks around a lake and through the hills of the hundred-acre sanitarium grounds. The most important rule for patients was to not talk about one's illness. There was no room for so-called self-pity at the "Muldoon's for women."[30]

The rise of physical culture and strenuous life movements at the turn of the century marked a cultural shift within the United States, wherein people stopped merely lamenting the loss of a romanticized, premodern, agrarian life and began trying to recreate aspects of its healthy ruggedness. If plowing row after mind-less row allowed farmers to strengthen their bodies and rest their brains, then calisthenics, bike riding, and basketball allowed urban Americans to do the same. Exercising simply for its own sake was inconvenient and could cost time and money, thereby making neurasthenia an important motivator, as it gave people the incentive of staying healthy. Further, with the growth of organiza-tions such as the YMCA and YWCA, as well as movements like physical cul-ture and "the strenuous life," Americans were less likely to see rest as the therapy for neurasthenia. "The traditional 'rest cure' . . . is being discarded by most physicians except in a special class of cases," the *New York Times* reported to readers in 1907; "The more modern remedy is known as the 'work cure.'"[31] Americans were not interested in becoming neurasthenics made soft by city life; they wanted to be robust, powerful people in the tradition of their rural forbears.

Handicrafts and Resort Living

The Arts and Crafts movement of the years around 1900 was one of the most conspicuous attempts to integrate tradition and authenticity into hectic, mod-ern lifestyles. Represented by persons such as John Ruskin and William Morris, the movement had originated in England during the second half of the nine-teenth century as an artistic response to what many considered the soulless, alienating manufacturing process of modern factories. Advocates encouraged people to learn traditional trades like bookbinding, pottery, and carpentry as a way of recapturing the sense of purpose that came from making something use-ful. Like physical culture, the Arts and Crafts movement represented an active alternative to the rest cures of the 1870s and by the 1890s, it had established itself as a therapeutic bastion against neurasthenia.[32]

For men and women worn out and driven to neurasthenia by the pressures of modern society, working with their hands proved therapeutic for rebuilding their lives. Congregationalist minister John Todd, an early advocate of handi-crafts in the United States and a contributor to Martin Luther Holbrook's health manual *Hygiene of the Brain and Nerves* (1878), suggested that "when you are weary at your writing table, when the brain reels or muddles, when the thoughts stagnate," then the time is right to start crafting manually. An amateur wood-worker, Todd claimed that a few hours dedicated to one's hobby would make the mind "refreshed and invigorated"; "I consider my workshop an invaluable aid to health." In 1904, Dr. Herbert James Hall founded a school of handicrafts (featuring pottery, weaving, woodcarving, and metal work) at Marblehead, Massachusetts, to provide occupational therapy for his neurasthenic patients at the nearby Devereux Mansion Sanitarium. "A practical school of Handcraft for neurasthenics has been my heart's desire for a number of years," he explained in a letter to Dr. Frederick Shattuck of Harvard. Hall argued that neurasthenia most often arose from debilitating effects of worry and anxiety, not from physical fatigue; thus the cure was to get patients to find hobbies that allowed them to forget their troubles, much as Sarah Butler Wister had done with her morning painting. For twenty-five dollars a week, neurasthenics could stay in a boarding house near the water, immerse themselves in nature, receive medical treatment, and restore their nerves in Hall's therapeutic workshop. Although funding was tight at first, soon the Devereux Mansion's workshop succeeded in marketing and selling patients' handcrafted products to help defray medical and educational costs. Hall's handiwork venture even attracted attention on the West Coast, with a 1908 article in the *Los Angeles Times* reporting that "Business and professional men who were on the verge of nervous breakdown have spent months working and been restored to health; and women with overwrought nerves have found that there was a cure in so simple a thing as working with the hands."[33] Arts and crafts were not as strenuous as the exercises at Muldoon's, but they were still a form of work cure requiring activity and concentration that redirected neurasthenic minds from their problems.

The idea that modern business persons should find relief producing traditional handicrafts possessed a certain poetic ring not lost on journalist Frank Marshall White. In 1910 White wrote a feature for *Outlook*, "The Occupation and Exercise Cure," in which his protagonist, referred to only as "the capitalist," was a millionaire corporate entrepreneur who looked and felt decades older than his actual forty-something years. Consulting with a nerve specialist, the capitalist complained of "inward trembling" characterized by "palpitation of the heart, poor sleep, occasional dizziness, pain in the back of the neck, difficulty in concentrating. . . , and, most of all, from various apprehensions, such as that of being about to fall, of losing [his] mind, of sudden death." The nerve specialist replied, "You present merely the ordinary signs of neurasthenia," explaining that the condition arose when people overused parts of the brain; relief could be found by changing lifestyles so that the overused parts of the brain could recuperate. "One of the best means to this end is manual occupation— drawing, designing, carpentry, metal-work, leather-work, weaving, basket making, bookbinding, clay-modeling, and the like—for in all these things the hands are kept busy, requiring concentration of attention, while new interests of an artistic and aesthetic nature are aroused." The idea of devoting his "trained intelligence, accustomed to cope with great problems of trade and finance" to "trivialities" such as basket weaving struck the capitalist as preposterous, but the nerve specialist charged a high fee for his services, so the capitalist, not wanting to squander the money nor the advice, followed along and enrolled in a handicraft resort in upstate New York. Much to his surprise and relief, after four months of basket weaving, book binding, and brass working, punctuated by tennis, golf, and fishing, the capitalist felt good enough to renew his high-powered corporate wrangling in New York City.[34]

White's semifictional account spoke to neurasthenia's reputation as an affluent illness. "Of course the institution that has been described is only for the well-to-do," White recognized, but he held out hope that the government and philanthropists could work together to make "occupation and exercise cures" available also to the poor. But one might suspect that "the capitalist" would not have found his basket weaving so therapeutic if he were forced to do it shoulder-to-shoulder with the nation's poor, as the exclusively high cost of his "cure" seemed just as efficacious as the act of weaving. Mitchell's exclusive and expensive private practice specializing in the rest cure employed a similar dynamic, wherein the cost of treatment not only created an expectation for success, but also provided an opportunity for conspicuous consumption.[35] The affluent could showed off their wealth by draping themselves in fine jewelry or wearing the most expensive suits; neurasthenia provided the opportunity to display economic power by participating in costly (but ostensibly therapeutic) hobbies.

It was often difficult to distinguish therapy from leisure. Indeed, for many people like "the capitalist," leisure away from the job *was* a therapy. A lingering Protestant work ethic made mainstream Americans wary of leisurely vacations. This presented a conundrum for would-be vacationers in the late nineteenth century: how could they enjoy leisure without violating their work ethic? One way the middle class resolved this dilemma was by making their vacations action-packed, event-driven excursions—leisure (since apart from the workplace), but not slothful (since active and busy).[36] White's article "The Occupation and Exercise Cure" and the case of homemaker turned vacationer Sarah Butler Wister demonstrate that neurasthenia offered another way to engage in restful leisure yet avoid accusations of sloth: call vacations therapeutic. "The capitalist" and Wister did not travel to arts and crafts resorts to *avoid* work so much as to recuperate so that they could *continue* to work.

Profit-driven resorts and sanitariums during the late nineteenth and early twentieth centuries encouraged Americans to avoid neurasthenia by distancing themselves from hectic city lives. For instance, the Mt. Clifton Resort, located two hours by train from Washington, D. C., in the mountains around Hedgesville, West Virginia, called itself a "First-Class place for those who are seeking health and rest." Brochures circulated throughout the East Coast vaunted Mt. Clifton's bass fishing, calming nature trails, and therapeutic, broad panoramic vistas, which reportedly helped people suffering from "wearied brain work and nervous exhaustion" caused by busy lives in claustrophobic cities. In Wrightsville Beach, North Carolina, the seaside New Tarrymoore Hotel sold itself to potential customers as a "wonderful health resort" where "weary bodies can but be made strong and active, and depressed minds can but be made bright and cheery." Not wanting to leave the public with the impression that Tarrymoore was a boring retreat for recovering invalids, brochures enticingly promoted it as a "veritable Pleasure Palace" of "gaiety and fashion": "At the hotel is found womanhood in its merriest mood and manhood in its handsomest appearance. . . . Wit sparkles brightly and laughter rings clear and true at this elegant seashore retreat."[37] Catering to exhausted parents as well as frisky teenagers, the Tarrymoore promised something for the entire family.

The link between health and leisure was particularly pronounced in promotional literature for western resorts. The Barker Hotel—the self-proclaimed "Gem of the Rockies!"—located in Manitou Springs, Colorado, targeted its brochures to two audiences: tourists and invalids. "Nowhere else can be found such a combination of conditions as unite to make this place the favorite resort of tourists and a veritable sanitarium for those in search of health," an 1885 hotel circular claimed. The dry alpine air and cool breezes combined with excursions through the mountains and resort activities to ensure that visitors "need never suffer from ennui."[38] The Loma Linda Sanitarium, located in Loma Linda, California, titled its 1900 brochure "For Health and Pleasure" and claimed that the landscape, climate, and natural surroundings of the turn-of-the-century San Bernardino Valley created an "ethereal trust for the purpose of comforting the weary, the lonely, the sick and distressed." Equipped with a sun parlor, an amusement building, medicated baths, massage facilities, faradic electrotherapy (for those who felt their energy running particularly low), central heating, electric lights, and a gourmet kitchen that produced delicious yet wholesome meals, Loma Linda sold itself as a "delightful spot for the over-worked business man to spend a few weeks . . . an Eden of repose for the nervous woman who seeks rest from the burdens of society, or the cares of the home . . . [and] an ideal spot for the modest pleasure seeker to enjoy the quiet charms of nature."[39] To ensure that weary neurasthenics frequented these resorts, prominent eastern physicians and western entrepreneurs formed collaborative relationships to help channel the affluent sick westward. For example, Santa Barbara's Miradero Sanitarium, founded by Dr. Philip King Brown on the California coastline, listed endorsements from such East Coast luminaries as Vincent Bowditch,

Frederick Shattuck, William Osler, and S. Weir Mitchell—all preeminent physicians in their fields.[40]

As 1900 approached, reference to neurasthenia began appearing in advertisements to boost land sales and migration to western states, especially California. For decades, boosters (mainly railroad companies, state governments, and chambers of commerce) had marketed land to tuberculosis victims on the premise that the dry climate and rural environment would help slow the illness. With Robert Koch's 1882 discovery of the *Mycobacterium tuberculosis* as the cause of the disease, it gradually went from being seen as a tragically romantic condition ("consumption") to being feared as a deadly contagion ("tuberculosis"). As the stigma of tuberculosis increased, land boosters stopped using it in promotional literature and began relying on neurasthenia as the new marketable illness to draw invalid investors west. The Southern California Bureau of Information stressed in 1892 how the region's fresh fruit and coastal air was particularly suited for those with "nervous complaints." The *Tourists' Guide Book to South California for the Traveler, Invalid, Pleasurist, and Home Seeker* (1894) claimed that the region offered "rest for the weary, recuperation for the overworked and restoration for the invalid." It was in Pasadena, California, a community founded on agriculture and affluent consumptives, that Charlotte Perkins Gilman found temporary relief from her neurasthenia in the late 1880s: "Everywhere there was beauty," she remembered years later in her autobiography, "and the nerve-rest of steady windless weather."[41]

The natural environment and salubrious climate that reportedly made rural sanitariums beneficial to health soon became commodities in themselves. In 1892, Charles Dudley Warner, a noted essayist and co-author with Mark Twain of *The Gilded Age* (1873), published *Our Italy*, an illustrated introduction to Southern California that celebrated the region's agricultural and therapeutic wonders. Protected by the Sierra Nevada range, deserts, and the Pacific Ocean, Southern California's invigorating climate remained cool (but never cold) and warm (but never hot) all year around. "Except a tidal wave from Japan, nothing would seem to be able to affect or disturb it," Warner claimed; "It goes without saying that this sort of climate would suit anyone in ordinary health, inviting and stimulating to constant out-of-door exercise, and that it would be equally favorable to that general break-down of the system which has the name of nervous prostration." Warner believed that there was no reason for Americans to travel abroad to Europe, traditionally *the* fashionable destination of wealthy American neurasthenics during the late nineteenth century: "Here is our Mediterranean! Here is our Italy!" Thanks to its "monotony of good weather" and its "perpetual bloom and color in orchards and gardens," Southern California even mimicked the Mediterranean's relaxed lifestyle that took away "nervousness and produce[d] a certain placidity, which might be taken for laziness by a Northern observer. . . . It is not unpleasant to think that there is a corner of the Union where there will be a little more leisure, a little more of serene waiting on Providence, an abatement of the restless rush and haste of our usual life."[42] Even in the 1890s, Southern California had a reputation for being laid-back. It was good for the nerves.

Nature and Recapturing the Frontier Spirit

Experiencing nature—being outdoors, breathing fresh air, hiking, hunting— emerged from the nineteenth century as key lifestyle antidotes for neurasthenia. The vital importance of nature had been a theme in some of the earliest writing on nervousness. Mitchell, well known for his rest cure, was also an early advocate of the "camp cure," which he originally suggested for neurasthenic men but later strongly urged for women as well, apologizing for his earlier oversight. Camping, a fact of life for previous generations of pioneers and frontier farmers, offered modern urbanites the opportunity to mimic the experiences of these hardy forebears and in the process reclaim from nature a degree of nervous energy. Camping also provided an inexpensive alternative to often expensive rural health resorts. After the initial investment of a wagon, tent, and basic equipment, an entire family could camp for the summer with only the cost of food. "All over our sparsely-inhabited land, places wild enough are within easy reach," Mitchell noted in 1888. He urged citizens of all incomes to turn to camping, "this peculiarly American mode" of recreation, as the healthy vacation choice. Hunting, fishing, hiking, rowing, photography, reading, and writing were all camp activities that exercised the mind and body, while immersion in nature afforded men and women solitude and the chance to escape the work and home pressures. "One gets near realities out of doors. . . . Thought is more sober; one becomes a better friend to one's self," Mitchell observed.[43] Nature allowed people to take stock of their lives, assess their priorities, and find health, happiness, and comfort.

For some Americans accustomed to the ways and habits of city life, the idea of camping for health was an absurdity. In 1878, a year after Mitchell first wrote of the "camp cure," *Scribner's* published a comical tale of an overworked husband and wife who, on the advice of their physician, decided to spend two weeks in September camping out next to a river a few miles from their house. "You need rest and change," their physician said; "Nothing will do you so much good as to camp out; that will be fifty times better than going to any summer resort. . . . Get a good tent and an outfit, be off to the woods, and forget all about business and domestic matters for a few weeks."[44] This modern couple were not experienced campers and their vacation turned into a nerve-wracking fiasco: they missed the ticking comfort of their clock; they were afraid of violent intruders and kept a gun nearby; they fretted over their house and frequently went home to make sure everything was in order; mosquitoes wreaked havoc; the fish did not bite; wind and rain nearly flooded them out; their neighbors did not understand why they were camping "for their health" and rumor spread that an epidemic was afoot, putting the entire town into panic. The story demonstrates how unusual it was during the 1870s for people willingly to give up civilized town comforts for rough conditions of outdoor life. If the campers were meant to represent typical townsfolk, then clearly the author thought much of America had lost touch with its hardy frontier traditions.

Neurasthenia gave Americans a reason to reacquaint themselves with their nation's frontier tradition. In 1885 Owen Wister Jr., the neurasthenic banker-turned-author son of Sarah Butler Wister, spent time roughing it in Medicine Bow, Wyoming, upon the medical advice of his uncle, the physician Mitchell. He kept a diary of his adventures and upon recovery used his experiences as inspiration for his genre-defining cowboy novel *The Virginian* (1902), which he dedicated to Theodore Roosevelt, his good friend who also ventured west to recover from his own bout of nervous exhaustion. Like many Americans at the time, Wister believed the west was a source of America's vital nervous energy, an energy that helped bring out the best in citizens, especially in Anglo-Saxon citizens. In an essay published by *Harper's* in 1895, Wister suggested that the west represented a borderland between civilized and uncivilized worlds that offered danger and opportunity in equal measures and awakened the energy and noble potential found within the Anglo-Saxon race. The western cowboy, Wister argued, was merely the latest phase in the social evolution of Anglo Saxons interacting with nature, an evolution tracing back to the days of Arthurian knights: "In personal daring and in skill as to the horse, the knight and the cowboy are nothing but the same Saxon on different environments . . . and no hoof in Sir Thomas Mallory shakes the crumbling plains with quadruped sound more valiant than the galloping that has echoed from the Rio Grande to the Big Horn Mountains." Living in the saddle out west offered cowboys "absolute health and strength," and made them, in the estimate of Wister, the ideal Americans, whose minds were kept sharp by the challenges they met and whose bodies were kept vital.[45]

By the 1890s, camping and outdoor life had become more widespread and stories documenting the salubrious effects of camping more commonly appeared in America's popular literature. In contrast to the ridiculous attempt at camping depicted in the *Scribner's* story, Robert Strahorn's 1896 "A Summer Outing on Northwestern Waters" made a therapeutic tour of the Rockies seem as normal as a tour of Europe. "Dick and I were fagged out. A rest was impera-tive," the story began. As regional heads of a large unnamed corporation, Strahorn and Dick had just guided their company through the latest "commercial cata-clysm" for which the 1890s were infamous. Breaking down under "years of strain such as few middle-age Americans live though," the two men listened to their doctors, who insisted they and their wives spend the entire summer camping in the Rocky Mountains, away from "telegraph, telephone, and locomotive," where "outdoor life was compulsory and isolation complete." With the help of hired guides, the foursome spent weeks fishing for rainbow trout, hunting deer, cooking in a Dutch oven, encountering bears, hiking from lake to lake, and living within the mountain forests. "Only the devotee of camp life knows the restfulness, luxury and healthfulness of a properly constructed 'odorous piney bed,'" Strahorn explained to readers. After weeks in the mountains, the campers emerged with "clear eyes, steady nerves and the strong strokes of rugged health."[46] This story helped normalize the idea of going camping not for the pure amusement of it—life was physically difficult and dangerous at times—so much as for the vitality of it. Months of bracing mountain air and rugged living compensated for years of enervating business life within America's modern, highly competitive corporate economy. The mountains represented a primitive but healthy existence presumably close to how nature intended people to live; business life represented a man-made overcivilization far removed from people's natural habitat.

Frederick Jackson Turner's seminal 1893 essay "The Significance of the Frontier in American History" brought additional attention to the energizing importance of undeveloped lands. The 1890 U.S. census had declared that a national territorial frontier no longer existed, meaning the era of pioneers and settlers was over and civilization had spread throughout the nation's borders. For Turner, a historian at the University of Wisconsin, this marked the "closing of a great historic movement" in which pioneers had struggled with nature, hewed their livelihoods out of the continent's vast forests, and developed an energetic personality that made the United States a singular nation. "To the frontier," Turner claimed, "the American intellect owes its striking characteris-tics," including "that coarseness and strength combined with acuteness and inquisitiveness; that practical, inventive turn of mind, quick to find expedients; that masterful grasp of material things, lacking in the artistic but powerful to effect great ends; that restless, nervous energy; that dominant individualism, working for good and for evil; and withal that buoyancy and exuberance which comes with freedom—these are traits of the frontier." Weaving a narrative rem-iniscent of Mitchell's romantic agrarianism as found in *Wear and Tear*, Turner argued that farmers' frontier experiences fueled the nation's industrial and eco-nomic development and provided the country with an egalitarian democratic tradition. "Energy, incessant activity," he contended in an essay on a similar topic, "became the lot of this new American."[47] For Turner, the key issue facing Americans going into the twentieth century was how they could preserve their energetic democratic tradition without the frontier experience. This question paralleled the conundrum at the heart of neurasthenia that Mitchell and Beard wrestled with: how were Americans going to have a healthy, productive future within the highly civilized society they had created?

Naturalist John Muir put forth an adamant answer: set aside natural parks and forests as places for city folk to frequent and replenish their nerves. Muir, a Scottish immigrant who had moved with his family to an Indiana farm when he was ten, saw the development of the modern city, with its stale air, cacoph-ony of noises, and constant movement as a dubious and debilitating phenome-non. "Our crude civilization engenders a multitude of wants," he reflected in his journal while camping among towering sequoias in the Sierra Nevada in 1875; "I chance to think of the thousands needing rest—the weary in soul and limb. . . . The hall and the theater and the church have been invented, and com-pulsory education. Why not add compulsory recreation? . . . Yet few think of pure rest or of the healing power of Nature."[48] Muir had a good point, and the presence of neurasthenia in American cities strengthened his argument. If the United States sought to ensure future generations of healthy and productive citizens, steps needed to be taken to offset the unhealthy anxiety and enervating activity of the city. If urban modern life was the source of neurasthenia, then, in Muir's opinion, the natural forests and mountain ranges were the obvious antidote.

In his remarkable life, Muir transformed himself from a wilderness tramp into the nation's leading environmentalist. With the help of Robert Underwood Johnson, a *Century Magazine* editor, Muir successfully lobbied to have Yosemite declared a National Park by Congress in 1890. In 1892 Muir founded the Sierra Club, dedicated to protecting the nation's natural habitats and encouraging urbanites to get out of the cities and experience nature.[49] By the early twentieth century, the desire to get back to nature was catching on: according to park records, approximately two-and-a-half thousand people visited Yosemite in 1885, over eight thousand in 1902, and over thirty-one thousand in 1915—a twelvefold increase in little over a generation. In his essay "The Wild Parks and Forest Reservations of the West," originally published in *The Atlantic* in 1898, Muir expressed delight to see Americans' appreciation for nature grow.

"Thousands of tired, nerve-shaken, over-civilized people are beginning to find out that going to the mountains is going home; that wildness is a necessity; and that mountain peaks and reservations are useful not only as fountains of timber but also fountains of life." This growing popular interest, Muir thought, needed to be encouraged to save urbanites from languishing in their busy cities "choked with care like clocks full of dust."[50] Muir did not suggest Americans give up their urban ways and modern lives, but he urged them to periodically reconnect with the earth to clear out the nervous tension that impaired their health, happiness, and comfort.

In his fight to protect wildlands, Muir found powerful allies among the nation's hunters and anglers. In December 1887, Teddy Roosevelt and George Bird Grinnell (who had founded the Audubon Society the previous year) gathered in Manhattan with a small group of outdoor enthusiasts from the elite ranks of New York society to found the Boone and Crockett Club, an organizational advocate for the exploration of America's wilderness, the establishment and enforcement of hunting regulations, and the conservation of forests, streams, and game.[51] Although Muir never hunted or even carried a gun in all his years hiking the Sierra Nevada, he was excited to enlist help in his fight to protect natural resources from exploitation, and he joined forces with the Boone and Crockett Club, which provided the insider political influence to pass conservation legislation while Muir and his naturalist colleagues helped shape public opinion. In what has been described as an elitist conspiracy, in 1891 they passed Section 24, an amendment to a general land law that gave the president authority to set aside public lands for preservation. Over the next decade, environmental advocates quietly worked through the White House to increase federal regulations on land use and to set aside thousands of acres for preservation, much to the chagrin of lumber, mining, and livestock industries. Once Roosevelt became president in 1901, the conservation of national parks and forests became part of the national agenda, and Boone and Crocket member Gifford Pinchot went about building the U. S. Forest Service into an independent, influential organization that dedicated itself to conserving the nation's natural resources and ensuring that future generations of Americans would be able to venture into a frontier-like environment to hike, camp, hunt, and, in the process, steel themselves for modern life. When President Roosevelt was in California in 1903 there was no question whom he would ask to be his personal guide through Yosemite: John Muir, who bought himself a poorly tailored yellow suit just for the occasion.[52]

As the early twentieth century approached and Americans became more familiar with neurasthenia, they took measures to manage the unhealthful effects of modern life with healthy activities. The speed with which the narrator of Marr's *Confessions of a Neurasthenic* changed lifestyles in search of health was farcical, but the fact that more and more people were making equivalent changes to their lives was reality. Schools were asking more from students, business was asking more from employees, social clubs and organizations were asking more from members, and even politics was asking more from politicians. The expectations placed upon modern Americans seemed to exceed their capacities, draining their energies and causing neurasthenia. The solution Americans developed was to balance the unhealthy with the wholesome so that they could retain their nervous energy, remain active, and avoid neurasthenia altogether. This became an issue of lifestyle, with people adopting new habits such as daily exercise, hobbies, rejuvenating vacations, and recreational camping, because these were practical, if not enjoyable, ways to avoid neurasthenia. That these activities continued to remain part of America long after neurasthenia faded from public memory speaks to their effectiveness in producing health, happiness, and comfort in ways that other treatments, such as electrotherapy and the rest cure, did not.

And despite its turn-of-the-century ubiquity, neurasthenia did fade. No specific germ was every identified as the definitive source for the disease, nor was the theory of nervous energy, upon which Beard had founded his diagnosis, ever proven. Consequently when changes began during the first few decades of the twentieth century that undermined the reciprocal cycle of neurasthenia information among physicians, patients, and popular culture, there was nothing to support the continued use of the diagnosis. Symptoms persisted, but by the 1920s they were less likely to be associated with neurasthenia.

Chapter 6

The Decline of Neurasthenia

"Nowadays," Dr. Peter Bassoe observed in 1927 to his colleagues of the Wisconsin State Medical Society, "among up-to-date physicians a diagnosis of neurasthenia is usually not well received." Bassoe went on to voice what many of his fellow physicians had already known for years: neurasthenia had outlasted its usefulness as a medical concept. "The term *neurasthenia* is a mile stone in the history of medicine, which at first marked progress but now impedes it," he explained to his audience, concluding that "while we should retain the useful ideas of the creators of the term, we had better drop the term itself."[1] Neurasthenia had a major run as one of America's most distinctive illnesses, but by the 1920s it was quickly losing the medical and cultural traction that had since 1869 made it such a successful way of understanding personal health.

That the neurasthenia diagnosis rapidly declined after 1920 might seem an unlikely scenario considering the nerve-wracking turmoil Americans experienced going into the decade. The nation's experience in the First World War exposed hundreds of thousands of American soldiers to machine guns, field artillery, trench warfare, and other horrors that caused grown men to become nervous wrecks. Then, as soldiers returned home after the war, they unwittingly brought with them a virulent and deadly strain of influenza that ran rampant through American communities, overwhelmed the nation's health services, and killed over half a million citizens. Amid this death, labor tensions exploded in 1919 as waves of strikes involving millions of workers paralyzed the American economy and shut down major cities such as Seattle, as well as entire industries—for instance, in the steel strike. By the end of that year,

Attorney General A. Mitchell Palmer was warning Americans that the country was on the precipice of a Bolshevik revolution, as a series of mail bombs and, later, an explosion on Wall Street that killed thirty-eight people whipped the nation into a frenzied fear that it might indeed fall into radical chaos. If there was ever a time when Americans might feel their nerves frayed, it was in 1920.

By that year, however, American medicine was in the process of overhauling its understanding of nervous disorders. The decision to move away from the neurasthenia diagnosis was a deliberate one on the part of doctors such as Bassoe who saw neurasthenia as an overly vague, cumbersome label; its protean quality might have attracted an earlier generation of doctors and helped build organized medicine, but by the twentieth century it had become a professional liability. The reciprocal cycle of information that allowed neurasthenia to thrive also meant that physicians had to share authority over symptoms with patients and advertisers, something the medical profession in the twentieth century wanted to avoid. In addition, the medical theory of nervous energy upon which Beard had predicated neurasthenia remained unproven and, in its place, doctors were developing new theories of health. These included chemical factors such as hormones and vitamins and, most important, psychic factors (as in psychiatry and psychology) that helped therapists reconceptualize symptoms of discomfort and unhappiness as the result of mental disorders rather than of exhaustion of nervous energy.

It took more than a change of opinion by doctors to cause neurasthenia to fall into decline and disuse as a concept within the United States. After all, neurasthenia was not just a medical diagnosis: it was also a way to advertise products, to understand one's spirituality, to critique gender roles, and to justify more leisurely activity and exercise. Changes in the way advertisers marketed health care products such as medicine also contributed to moving the public discourse away from neurasthenia, as Americans were no longer bombarded with promotions seeking to education them about neurasthenia. As the medical professional made the move to marginalize the neurasthenia diagnosis and advertisers changed the way they marketed health care products, the term itself faded but comfort and happiness remained as hallmarks of good health.

Medical Reform, Hormones, and Vitamins

Since the neurasthenia diagnosis typically denoted a group of symptoms rather than a provable etiology, there was little consensus going into the twentieth century as to what the diagnosis actually stood for. Speaking in front of the Ontario Medical Association in 1905, a frustrated William Pritchard from New York called the neurasthenia diagnosis a "phantom, once a tree, now a forest and rapidly becoming a wilderness, so rank and riotous is its growth." He found that over the thirty-five years since its initiation, the neurasthenia diagnosis had been so "elaborated and broadened and abused that to-day it means almost anything and with equal truth almost nothing." Pritchard was by no means alone in his assessment. John Donley estimated in 1906 that "there is no word used in medicine which has been so loosely and withal so vaguely applied as this very word, 'neurasthenic.'" Ten years later, Dr. Robert Morris pointed out in his health guide *Doctors Versus Folks* that the diagnosis no longer had universal meaning, as each branch of medicine understood it through the lens of its own specialty. Surgeons, for instance, understood neurasthenia to be the result of sick organs that needed to be removed, psychiatrists interpreted the condition as the result of a maladjusted psyche in need of calibration, neurologists believed it the product of poor nerve tone that might require tonics, and hygienists saw it as the result of a poor diet or lack of exercise.[2] The diagnosis had essentially become an exercise in word play, with doctors, psychologists, and "mind curists" all having different languages to describe the same symptomatic phenomena.

The vague nature of neurasthenia conflicted with changes happening within the American medical profession at the turn of the twentieth century. The American Medical Association reorganized itself in 1901 and assumed broad regulatory power aimed at marginalizing practitioners who did not fit its model of scientific medicine. A few years before, the establishment of Johns Hopkins Medical School in 1893 revolutionized medical education within the United States by emphasizing laboratory science and clinical experience, developments that the Carnegie Foundation's Flexner Report capitalized on in 1910 in seeking to establish a standardized medical school curriculum that stressed the "science" over the "art" of medicine. As a result, twentieth-century physicians began to expect a great deal more specificity in diagnoses and more authority over symptoms than had their nineteenth-century colleagues. Diagnoses built upon a defined pathology were given preference over those predicated on a vague theory. Neurasthenia, a condition with an unproven concept of "nervous energy" taken on faith for decades, seemed hopelessly antiquated to this new generation of physicians. Instead of neurasthenia, doctors in the twentieth century increasingly relied on more specific explanations of health (including hormones, vitamins, and psychiatric and psychological factors) to describe Americans' unhappiness and discomfort.

The 1902 discovery of hormones began the process of parsing the neurasthenia diagnosis and allowing physicians to speak about health in a more specific, scientifically based manner. The term *hormone* had existed since the days of Hippocrates to denote an essential life force, but it was British physiologists William M. Bayliss and Ernest H. Starling who first used it in its modern sense to describe glandular secretions that influenced bodily function. Their adoption of the age-old term *hormone* reflected the belief that they had stumbled upon the chemical equivalent of life force. In less than a decade, physicians in the United States were attributing all sorts of symptoms previously associated with neurasthenia, especially gastrointestinal issues such as constipation and diarrhea, to hormone function. Douglas VanderHoof of Richmond's Memorial Hospital explained to his colleagues that hormones represented "chemical messengers" responsible for the smooth functioning of bodily organs and, if hormone secretion was abnormal, so too would be the function of the body's affected organs.[3] The causal agent was different from that of neurasthenia's theory of nervous energy, but the hormonal concept still provided a systemic understanding of bodily health by which dissimilar symptoms, from lethargy to indigestion to mood swings, could all be traced to organic imbalances.

Physicians found it easy to superimpose the theory of hormone function overtop the theory of nervous energy. For instance, Max Schlapp, professor of neuropathology at Cornell University Medical College, gave a series of lectures in 1911 on "modern women" and their role in the supposed racial degeneration of America, a well-rehearsed topic addressed by neurasthenia experts Beard and Mitchell since the 1870s. Schlapp told the usual story of how modern women overtaxed their supply of "nerve energy," but updated his claim by arguing that low nervous energy led to lower production levels of hormones. As reported by the *New York Times* (whose science writer struggled with the spelling of "hormones," calling them "harmons"), Schlapp did not account for growing rates of crime, insanity, and feeblemindedness among children in the "usual way" by citing poverty and broken homes, but rather attributed these to what babies did not get from their parents: "a sufficient amount of 'harmons' to mass healthy cells into brain centres."[4] Schlapp may have been running fast and loose with the concept of hormones, but his talk demonstrates how easy it was for new ideas coming out of early twentieth-century laboratories to be grafted onto the older discourses from America's experience with neurasthenia, even inheriting their sexist premises.

Learning how to control hormonal imbalances seemed an ideal way of ensuring personal health. In a 1920 essay, "On Prolonging Human Life," Dr. Eugene Lyman Fisk argued that hormonal function was the key to the physical and mental vigor necessary for longevity and happiness. "Excess or deficiency of hormones may cause profound changes not only in physical condition, but in character and personality," he explained to readers of the

North American Review. Mimicking the giddy optimism that Beard had held for the study of nervous energy fifty years before, Fisk boldly claimed that hormones contained the secret that would someday provide immortality. "The many examples of profound physical and psychic changes resulting from variation in the supply of hormones," he reasoned, "will enable us to administer combinations of substances that will maintain life and health indefinitely." The implications were radical, according to Fisk, as they indicated the next stage in social evolution, wherein people would be allowed "alternative destinies" from which to choose.[5] Such claims reflected medical science's fickle nature and how a new discovery could so quickly infatuate physicians and marginalize stale and unproven concepts such as neurasthenia.

Vitamins represented another scientific discovery that worked to displace the neurasthenia diagnosis. Polish biochemist Kazimierz Funk first coined the term *vitamin* in 1912 to label a vital ingredient in food that he could isolate in the laboratory. The scientific medical community quickly began attributing specific diseases such as scurvy, beriberi, and pellagra to vitamin deficiencies, and speculated on a host of symptoms that might also be related to vitamin deficiencies. An article in the *American Journal of the Medical Sciences* faulted vitamin deficiencies for loss of appetite, "general weakness," and sickly babies, all symptoms that a generation earlier could have easily been attributed to neurasthenia. By 1920 it was not unusual to see vitamins referred to as a universal source of health in much the same way that nineteenth-century physicians had described nervous energy. A 1919 article in the *Indiana Farmer's Guide*, for instance, celebrated vitamins as the "true life and strength-giving qualities of food" thereby making corn silage, reportedly chock full of vitamins, the ultimate food upon which to fatten cattle and cultivate enriched beef for the American consumer.[6]

The discussion of the universal importance of vitamins included popular sources as well as medical and farm journals. In 1917 the *New York Times* stressed the need for women to have up-to-date scientific knowledge so that they could more effectively feed their families healthy meals. "Modern housekeeping demands a knowledge of a balanced ration and food value," the *Times* reported, "with a new vocabulary including 'vitamins,' 'calories,' and other words full of meaning." The twentieth-century housewife no longer was being coached on how to preserve the nervous energy of her family; instead she was taught to efficiently manage health through the kitchen and to use domestic science to record vitamins and caloric energy. Even patent medicine manufacturers realized the importance of updating their advertising to incorporate the latest in health research. Panopepton, a product made from fortified beef extract, was advertised in 1919 as being full of "gastric and pancreas enzymes . . . , carbohydrates, proteins, amino-acids, [and] vitamins." Simply using the new language of metabolic and digestive health gave Panopepton a veneer of scientific credibility. It is hardly surprising that one of the first generation of multivitamin tablets, One-A-Day, was produced in 1940 by Miles Laboratories, the twentieth-century name of Miles Medical Company, to supplement the company's bottom line while sales for its supposedly nervous-energy-rich neurasthenia cure, Nervine, decreased.[7] Scientifically proven and easy to understand as the nutritional component of healthy food, by 1920 vitamins, along with hormones, were conceptually supplanting nervous energy (and therefore neurasthenia) in the minds of Americans.

Rise of Psychiatric and Psychological Explanations

The discovery of hormones and vitamins provided alternative ways to explain neurasthenic symptoms, but the most important therapeutic development of the twentieth century responsible for the decline of the neurasthenia diagnosis occurred in the intrapsychic disciplines of psychiatry and psychology. Much of the impetus for this came from New Thought, out of which had developed the spiritual "mind cures" advocated by writers such as Horatio Dresser and administered in a more organized fashion by Christian Scientists and the Emmanuel movement. James Jackson Putnam recognized the effectiveness of these mind cures in 1895 in his article "Psychical Treatment of Neurasthenia," and his Harvard colleague William James acknowledged their therapeutic usefulness in *The Varieties of Religious Experience* (1902). Neither Putnam nor James argued for the elimination of the neurasthenia diagnosis; they only sought to have fellow physicians recognize the potential usefulness of incorporating psychological techniques, especially suggestion, into regular medicine. Within a decade of Putnam's paper, a number of physicians began advocating for more drastic action, calling for neurasthenia's diagnostic retirement in favor of an illness nomenclature more closely associated with developments in psychiatry and psychology.[8]

Cornell neurologist Charles L. Dana began this process in 1904 with a paper read before the Boston Society of Psychiatry and Neurology, "The Partial Passing of Neurasthenia," which he published in the *Boston Medical and Surgical Journal* that same year. A generation younger than S. Weir Mitchell and George M. Beard, Dana was a mainstay within America's neurological community that had developed in conjunction with the neurasthenia diagnosis. In his paper, Dana argued that psychiatry, built upon new research coming out of Europe by people such as Emil Kraepelin, had undergone a "renaissance" that "aroused deeply the interest and respect of neurologists to whom for many years alienism has stood chiefly for politics and stewardship."[9] He was cognizant of the historic tension between neurologists and psychiatrists, which traced back to the initial rise of the neurasthenia diagnosis during the 1870s and 1880s, but Dana believed that by 1904 psychiatry had reinvented itself to become the cutting edge of American as well as European medicine. He was willing to sacrifice the neurasthenia diagnosis in the hope of securing a rapprochement between neurology and psychiatry as a way of improving professional medical care.

In "The Partial Passing of Neurasthenia," Dana estimated that half of all neurasthenia cases could be traced to some sort of localized physical condition, while the other half were the result of mental illness that warranted psychiatric treatment. "If one follows it up very closely," he told his audience and readers, "we may yet end in finding that there is no such thing as neurasthenia at all." He recast neurasthenia as an "understudy of some particular type of insanity, or . . . the forming stage of some major psychosis" rather than an independent diagnosis resulting from lack of nervous energy. Dana was aware of the popular stigma attached to psychiatric mental disorders—the neurasthenia diagnosis itself developed largely out of the late nineteenth-century backlash against asylum care and all things "insane"—but he hoped to cultivate a diagnostic middle ground between mental health and insanity that would prove acceptable to both doctors and patients. To this end, he suggested making *phrenasthenia* a new diagnostic category—an obvious play on *neurasthenia* but linked to weakness in the mind (*phren-*) rather than in the nervous system (*neur-*). As proof of neurasthenia's mental origin, he drew attention to the plethora of mind cures administered by physicians and nonphysicians alike, arguing, as Putnam did nine years earlier, that their success testified to the condition's psychological nature.[10]

Dana's attempt to bridge the professional differences between neurology and psychiatry yielded some success, as psychiatrists were quick to support his call to move away from the neurasthenia diagnosis in favor of a nomenclature coming from mental therapeutics. In 1905, psychiatrist Alder Blumer appeared before the Boston Society of Psychiatry and Neurology to issue Dana a rejoinder titled "The Coming of Psychasthenia," later published in the *Journal of Nervous and Mental Disease*. He thanked Dana for "so large and important a concession of territory" ceded by neurology to psychiatry, and estimated that Dana had effectively staved off a renewed professional war between "militant" neurologists and psychiatrists over neurasthenia and the patients associated with it. Citing medical work by French psychiatrist Pierre Janet, Blumer suggested using the term *psychasthenia*, rather than *phrenasthenia*, to denote mental-based neurasthenia cases; while the two were essentially equivalents, Blumer argued that leaders in the field of psychoneurosis favored the former.[11]

Like Dana, Blumer was of a younger generation than those psychiatrists and neurologists who bickered during the 1870s and 1880s, and he was interested in closer relations between the two fields. Nonetheless he was still bothered by what he believed were decades of neurologists' "incursions ever and anon into the debatable territory of the psychiatrists." Blumer recognized that, historically, psychiatrists were stigmatized by the lunatic asylum and were not trusted by the American people, so that when E. H. Van Deusen first introduced the concept of neurasthenia, people avoided using it. Neurologists, especially Beard, had saved the diagnosis, Blumer admitted, by repackaging it as a fashionable illness and making it a "household word," a tribute to the neurologists' promotional savvy and ability to give "morbid states pleasing appellations" that attracted patients.[12] From Blumer's perspective, that is, Dana had brought neurasthenia back home to psychiatry and neurologists should be appreciated for doing what psychiatrists could not: forging a sizeable medical market out of the unhappiness and discomfort associated with the condition.

Now back in possession of the neurasthenia diagnosis, followers of psychiatric medicine—who by this time included many neurologist converts—were eager to dismantle the diagnosis and use new theories of the mind to reinterpret neurasthenic symptoms. In 1906 John E. Donley, the physician of nervous diseases at St. Joseph's Hospital in Providence, Rhode Island, argued in the newly founded *Journal of Abnormal Psychology* that psychological theories coming out of Europe by people such as Joseph Grassett, Janet, Josef Breuer, and Sigmund Freud and championed by Americans such as James Jackson Putnam, Morton Prince, and Boris Sidis pointed the way for reconceptualizing neurasthenia as the disintegration of personality. He defined personality as "that living, unitary, self-conscious, mind-body mechanism which brings us in relation with the outer world of men and things and which we call 'myself.'" Personality acted as a mental health regulator, according to Donley, that allowed a person to withstand the challenges posed by physical adversity (metabolic problems, toxins, organ disturbances) or emotional adversity (terror, fear, anxiety); over time, physical and mental challenges could wear down personality, causing the amplification of unhappiness and discomfort until a person could no longer function properly.[13] Reframed this way, the path to good health went through one's personality—one's consciousness—rather than one's nervous system.

Donley recognized the need to treat the body when wear and tear was responsible for weakening the personality—insomniacs needed to sleep, for instance—but he stressed the role of mental therapy in healing so-called neurasthenics. He gave an example of a clergyman, a patient of his, who overworked himself into a neurasthenic breakdown characterized by a foreboding of doom. Despite his fears, the clergyman accepted an invitation to dinner, during which he "suffered from dizziness, flushings, and a general feeling of instability, while his obsessions and fears swooped down upon him." What saved him, according to Donley, was the recognition that his sickness was simply the result of a weakened personality, a realization that temporarily gave him the self-control to "stick it out and to present a solid front to his obsessions, fears, and other sensations."[14] With psychological methods such as this, the power for improvement lay with patients themselves, and physicians acted as guides rather than as administrators of medical procedures such as electrotherapy or the rest cure. In this way, Donley's psychological understanding of neurasthenia echoed the self-help quality of Horatio Dresser's New Thought writings and Susan Elizabeth Blow's therapeutic spiritual philosophy, both of which focused on the ability of the mind to fortify and heal itself.

Like others who advocated a mental reinterpretation of neurasthenia, Donley was self-conscious that his message might be understood as an endorsement of New Thought and Christian Science mind cures. "The mere enunciation of such a theory [that neurasthenia represented the disintegration of personality] may possibly appear to many to be unduly novel and to savor strongly of metaphysics," he admitted to readers. Dana, too, was cognizant of how close psychiatric mental therapeutics resembled spiritualist mind cures, remarking that he ran "the risk of having Mrs. Eddy claim me for her own." Since the 1890s, the medical profession had been concerned with the success that Christian Science and New Thought practitioners had been having treating neurasthenia cases, and the development of the Emmanuel Movement in 1906 further threatened to blur the boundaries between professional medicine and spiritual mind cures. It was a tall order for physicians such as Putnam, Dana, Blumer, and Donley to co-opt the effective elements of New Thought mind cures and bring them into the community of professional medicine during that community's process of reorganizing itself along more strictly scientific lines, a process highly suspicious of anything that smacked of faith healing. A new language needed to be established that was more or less consistent with scientific medicine and did not borrow excessively from New Thought, yet could communicate many of the same processes that took place in nineteenth-century mind cures.

It was an Austrian physician, Sigmund Freud, whose systematic theories of the mind helped provide a therapeutic language that further redefined neurasthenic symptoms as products of mental health rather than of lack of nervous energy. Trained in Vienna as a neurologist, Freud began identifying the psychosomatic roots of illness in the 1880s, at first utilizing hypnotism in treatments but then moving on to what he called his "talk cure" (later known as *psychoanalysis*) to help people regain health by resolving issues repressed in their minds. During this time, American physicians were distancing themselves from formal talk cures, associating them with the mind-cure movement so long championed by rivals within Christian Science and New Thought. By the time American physicians began taking mind cures seriously, at the start of the twentieth century, Freud's theories were comparatively developed, richly detailed with case studies, and built around a seemingly scientific understanding of the mind. This combination proved compelling for American physicians newly organized around the concept of scientific medicine and seeking an alternative to the musty neurasthenia diagnosis.

Although a handful of American physicians and scholars had encountered Freud through his German-language publications, it was not until 1909 that the Austrian neurologist began to seriously influence the way Americans understood mental health. That year, psychologist G. Stanley Hall invited Freud to travel to the United States to give a series of lectures at Clark University, where Hall was president. In the opinion of Hall, as well as of other eminent authorities on the mind, such as Putnam and Ernst Jones, America needed the presence of someone like Freud to act as a catalyst to help shape the developing psychotherapy movement—professional medicine's brand of mind cure— within American medicine. In 1908, Putnam and others sought to establish a place for psychotherapy within the orbit of scientific medicine with the launching of the *Psychotherapy* series of readers. The next year, the *Journal of Nervous and Mental Disease* further expanded the available information on psychotherapy by publishing a compilation of Freud's essays translated for the American market, where people were eager to learn what they could of his psychoanalytic theories.[15] It was this edited compilation that introduced to the English-speaking world Freud's opinions on neurasthenia.

In an article titled "On the Right to Separate from Neurasthenia a Definite Symptom-Complex as 'Anxiety Neurosis,'" Freud sought to peel away a large portion of the neurasthenic diagnosis in favor of a psychological understanding of illness. Originally published in German in 1895, then translated into English in 1909, Freud's article argued that many so-called neurasthenics actually suffered from a condition he called *anxiety neurosis*, characterized by general irritability, feelings of doom, anxiety attacks, insomnia, vertigo, phobias, susceptibility to pain, and diarrhea—many of the classic symptoms that

originally drew people to the neurasthenia diagnosis. Although Freud acknowledged that some of these cases may have arisen from battling a severe illness or
overwork, he believed the most common cause of anxiety neurosis was sexual
apprehension, which he traced to the fears men and women had concerning
sexual performance, as well as the loss of sexual satisfaction caused by coitus
interruptus or the cessation of habitual masturbation.[16] Linking health concerns
to sexual behavior was nothing new—male patients at the Cooper medical
clinic, for instance, often associated their neurasthenia with sex—but to do
so in such a deliberate and systematic way as did Freud marked a new era in
medicine.

Within a few years of Freud's 1909 visit, the United States had a growing
community of practitioners dedicated to his premise of mental health and the
promise of psychotherapy. Publications such as the *Journal of Nervous and
Mental Disease* and the newly founded *Journal of Abnormal Psychology*
helped generate a professional dialogue on psychotherapy that steadily shifted
attention away from neurasthenia and its physiologically based treatments
(such as Mitchell's rest cure and Beard's electrotherapy) toward the potential
benefit of specialist-led mind cures. Psychotherapy was not a standardized
movement, as Donley recognized in 1911 when he observed that it "can have
no definite, clear-cut boundaries," and that "what we include to-day in the psychotherapeutic armory we may . . . exclude tomorrow." The treatment strategy
was broadly defined and pragmatic, characteristics it shared with the neurasthenia diagnosis, and would exist on the margins of the American Medical
Association's vision of scientific medicine in the decades that followed.

Psychotherapy redefined health away from the paradigm of nervous
energy, upon which neurasthenia stood, toward a new psychological paradigm.
Without faith in the existence of nervous energy, neurasthenia became a term
of convenience that denoted a recognizable group of symptoms but lacked
a proven scientific basis. People continued to employ the diagnosis in a psychotherapeutic context alongside mention of neuroses and psychoses, but
neurasthenia's influence on American medicine was clearly fading and would
soon disappear altogether, with discussion of neuroses and psychoses taking
its place.[17]

The First World War and the recognition of shell shock accelerated the
linguistic handoff between neurasthenia and psychological ways of describing
health. On the surface, shell shock looked consistent with neurasthenia: they
shared similar symptoms of fatigue, irritability, headaches, inability to concentrate, and inability to act; and both could occur even if no obvious physical
trauma took place. This prompted military physicians on both sides of the

Atlantic to routinely use the term *neurasthenia* to describe affected soldiers. This shell shock neurasthenia, however, was understood as a primarily psychological phenomenon rather than as the result of an impaired nervous system. Colonel Pearce Bailey, chief of the Division of Neurology and Psychiatry in the surgeon general's office, defined shell shock in 1918 as a "war neurosis . . . a personal reaction to a military situation," and attributed soldiers' "nervousness" to their neuroses rather than to a weakened nervous system (as physicians would have done a generation earlier). The very term *shell shock* upset Bailey, who believed it gave the mistaken impression that an organic condition existed, rather than a functional mental disorder treatable by psychotherapy. Neurasthenia had a place in his description of shell shock, but in a supportive role alongside psychasthenia to describe a specific type of shell shock ("neuroses of neurasthenic or psychasthenic type"), which severed neurasthenia from its neurological foundations and further whittled away what was once an encompassing, prodigious diagnosis.[18]

Aside from the growing influence of psychotherapy at the eve of the war, there were other reasons why American physicians such as Bailey privileged a psychological understanding of shell shock. As a military physician and representative of the surgeon general's office, Bailey was concerned about the financial burden if the government had to dispense "favorable pensions" to shell-shocked soldiers, whom he estimated to comprise about 10 percent of total casualties. In his opinion, psychological injuries could be cured effectively through psychotherapies that employed the power of suggestion, thus allowing the federal government to save money by investing in temporary psychological treatment rather than paying out lifetime disability pensions as it would to those with crippling physical injuries.

Another reason why American physicians emphasized the role of psychological neuroses over neurasthenia in shell shock was because they leaned heavily on the shell shock work of British experts, whose nation had been fighting for nearly three years before American soldiers entered the conflict. British psychologist Charles Samuel Myers first coined the term *shell shock* in 1915 and used the language of his discipline to define it. In addition, neurasthenia ("the American disease") never exerted as much influence on British medicine as it did on American, and, although they referenced neurasthenia, there was little impetus for British researchers to incorporate neurasthenia as a major factor in shock cases, preferring instead to rely on psychological models they were accustomed to using. Consequently, when organizations such as the American Medical Association published digests of shell shock research, British sources were well represented but neurasthenia was not.[19]

American newspapers kept readers abreast of the latest medical developments concerning shell shock, and, in the process, telegraphed the shifting status of neurasthenia within the medical community to the population at large. The *New York Times Magazine*, for instance, ran a 1918 feature on shell shock and Smith College's decision to provide "war emergency summer school" as part of a program to train nurses to care for what was expected to be a large influx of shell-shocked soldiers needing care. Quoting psychiatrist L. Pierce Clark, the article described shell shock as "any bad case of nervous disorganization directly brought on as a result of participation in the war," and further went on to use both *neurasthenia* and *neurosis* as *shell shock* synonyms. Participating Smith students would take two months of classes in psychology, sociology, mental psychiatry, occupational therapy, military usage, and record writing—but no neurology.[20] Readers would have had little doubt that shell shock, and by association neurasthenia, formed a psychological condition in need of psychiatric medicine.

Understood as a psychological condition, neurasthenia could not long continue as an active diagnosis because the language of neuroses and psychoses made the diagnosis redundant at best and confusingly counterproductive at worst. When neurasthenia's slide toward psychology is seen alongside the discovery of vitamins and hormones, the diagnosis was in clear decline and needed to be retired. Such was the conclusion of a 1925 Veterans Bureau study that found that men previously diagnosed with neurasthenia were actually suffering from an assortment of physical problems, including tuberculosis, endocrine disturbances, digestive disorders, and focal infections, as well as mental problems such as early psychosis, nocturnal epilepsy, and constitutional psychopathies. "This one diagnosis," the report said about neurasthenia, "has been allotted greater use and greater abuse than any other diagnosis known." Unequivocal in his conclusion, the report's author stated: "It is my opinion that the diagnosis of neurasthenia has served its purpose, outlived its usefulness, and could at this time be left out of the nomenclature."[21] Disenchanted with a diagnosis based on the unproven concept of nervous energy, America's medical establishment by 1920 had put into full swing the process of parsing neurasthenia into more specific physiological and psychological conditions, soon rendering the diagnosis a medical relic, once too influential to simply disappear but lacking the credibility to be taken seriously by twentieth-century scientific medicine.

Phasing out the neurasthenia diagnosis not only allowed for the development of more specific diagnoses, it also allowed physicians a greater level of professional authority over health issues. For years, critics of neurasthenia argued that the disease's popularization encouraged patients to pressure physicians into issuing the diagnosis without a thorough examination. In 1894, for instance, the vice president of the American Medical Association, I. N. Love, estimated that 90 percent of neurasthenia cases were "spurious" and the product of patients who bullied physicians into bequeathing the recognizable diagnosis. This negotiated diagnostic process was a product of neurasthenia's reciprocal cycle of information that allowed physicians, patients, and popular culture alike to share authority over the disease. By moving away from the discussion of neurasthenia and toward other conditions not yet popularized, such as hormone imbalances, vitamin deficiencies, neuroses, and psychoses, physicians reduced patients' ability to partake in the diagnostic process, and in the process claimed greater professional control over neurasthenic symptoms. To an extent, this made the parsing of the neurasthenia diagnosis a necessary part of the American Medical Association's drive to further professionalize physicians' authority over medical issues.[22]

Crackdown on Drug Advertising

As a popularized condition, neurasthenia owed its success as a diagnosis to more than just America's physicians and patients. In particular, the nation's pharmaceutical companies printed millions of circulars and advertising handbills to increase their sales by encouraging people to self-diagnose neurasthenia and to self-medicate. Given neurasthenia's broad range of symptoms, it proved a most lucrative diagnosis for drug companies to promote, and thus, even if professional physicians were to phase out the diagnosis, aggressive drug advertising alone would have been sufficient to keep neurasthenia an active part of everyday Americans' vocabulary regarding health, happiness, and comfort. Professional physicians did not allow this to happen, however, and, in its mission to secure its authority over medical issues, the American Medical Association embarked on what became a successful campaign to limit pharmaceutical advertising, which in turn reduced neurasthenia's popularization by keeping mention of the condition out of public view.

Targeting what it called "secret nostrums," in 1900 the American Medical Association (AMA) asserted the right to deny advertising space within its journal to any proprietary medicine that did not follow new AMA guidelines aimed at eliminating "charlatanism, deception, and quackery" within the drug industry. If companies wanted a presence within the pages of the *Journal*, and therefore tacit Association endorsement, they had to make their medicine's formula available to the AMA for review and eliminate any advertised claim of their product being a "cure-all." This was a bold move on the AMA's part, as one study at the time estimated medicine companies were capitalized at $250 million and spent a greater percentage of their worth on advertising than did any other industry on earth, meaning any decision to forego medicine advertising would have serious economic repercussions. During the first year of the campaign, the *Journal of the American Medical Association* paid a financial price and lost over $8,000 in advertising revenue, but it remained adamant that it would continue its boycott against advertising of proprietary medicine and would serve as a model for other journals and newspapers. This determination turned out short-lived, as reorganization in 1901 redirected the AMA's attention to bureaucratic matters, causing the antiproprietary-medicine campaign to lose focus while proprietary medicine manufacturers continued to use their immense budgets to saturate the nation's medical and popular press with advertising.[23]

It took the efforts of muckraking journalists, most notably Samuel Hopkins Adams, to turn popular opinion against proprietary medicines and create a national environment conducive to regulating drug advertising. Beginning in late 1905, Adams, an investigative medical journalist, wrote a series of damning articles for *Collier's Weekly* titled "The Great American Fraud," in which he set out to give a "full explanation and exposure of patent-medicine methods, and the harm done to the public by this industry," which he argued was "founded on fraud and poison." Adams documented deaths caused by proprietary medicines and revealed their addictive levels of alcohol, cocaine, and opiates. He took medicine advertising to task for being misleading and a public nuisance, and argued that self-diagnosis and self-medication was a dangerously manipulative practice that ruined lives and broke apart families. Recognizing the importance of having public opinion on their side in the debate over proprietary medicines, the AMA funded a large-scale reprinting of a bound edition of Adams's *Great American Fraud* and distributed it throughout the nation to further stoke popular resentment toward patent medicine producers.[24] Despite the size of their advertising budgets, pharmaceutical companies were in retreat and needed to refurbish their image and regain the public's trust.

The AMA kept up the pressure on medicine manufacturers and their advertising methods by establishing, in 1905, the Council on Pharmacy and Chemistry, a regulatory agency within the association that was designed to evaluate and certify medicines produced by industry. The council used the expert opinions and laboratory resources available to the AMA and issued a set of ten rules that medicine companies had to follow to earn AMA approval and inclusion in the publication *New and Non-Official Remedies* published by the *Journal of the American Medical Association*.[25] Medicines that did not follow

the outlined rules received no AMA endorsement, were shunned by physicians, and were publicly shamed for not meeting the minimum standards of
health and responsibility set forth by the AMA, which by this time was cement-
ing its reputation as the nation's foremost authority on health matters.

Two of the new AMA rules governing medicines had a dramatic effect on
neurasthenia's popularized status by limiting the ability of medicine advertisers to use the neurasthenia diagnosis to sell products. One rule forbade a medicine from being advertised directly to the public, which helped reduce the
numerous marketing circulars that in previous decades had helped bring the
neurasthenia diagnosis to public attention. Another rule forbade a medicine
from having any diagnosis mentioned on its packaging or accompanying literature, which limited the ability of manufacturers to associate their medicines
with a particular illness, such as neurasthenia.[26] Taken together, these new AMA
guidelines sought to limit drug companies' ability to distribute medical information that might encourage the public to self-diagnosis and self-medicate,
a marketing strategy that had generated profits by getting people to think of
themselves as sick with neurasthenia, among other illnesses. Absent wide-
spread self-diagnosis, Americans had to rely more heavily on the diagnostic
opinions of professional physicians, a group in the process of abandoning the
neurasthenia label altogether.

A medicine company could ignore the AMA's new rules, but this came at
a risk to their reputation that could have a dramatic influence on a company's
legal rights, as the case of Miles Medical Company vs. The May Drug Company
demonstrated in early 1906. Sensitive to the retail price of its products, Miles
Medical, creators of Nervine and advertisements that helped popularize
neurasthenia, routinely had retailers enter into contracts agreeing not to sell
their proprietary medicines for less than the price listed on the packaging.
When the May Drug Company, a discount drug store in Pittsburgh, cut the price
of Miles Medical products on its shelves and claimed that pricing contracts
constituted an illegal restraint of trade, the pharmaceutical company took the
drug store to court, claiming that the discounting of Miles products cheapened
its brand, which the company had spent about $2 million in advertising to
establish.[27]

After hearing the case, Judge James R. Macfarlane announced that, even
though Miles Medical won their legal argument, he could not in good conscience
rule in favor of Miles Medical. The reason: their marketing of secret-formula
proprietary medicines represented a "serious menace" to the "health and lives
of the public." In his written opinion, Macfarlane denounced Miles Medical's
strategy of using the mail to prescribe medicine as fraudulent, and called the

company's attempt to have people self-diagnose and self-medicate the "height of folly" and "contrary to public policy."[28] This was a powerful rebuke of Miles Medical Company and proprietary medicine producers as a whole, as the field's shady reputation and seemingly unscrupulous advertising essentially stripped the company of its legal rights and ability to seek redress using the court system. The solution to this problem was not simply more advertising; the patent medicine industry had to rebuild its reputation by fundamentally changing the way it did business and ally itself with the AMA, which required changes in advertising, changes that would take mention of neurasthenia out of the public eye.

Federal and state regulation of proprietary medicines increased from 1906 onward. In response to public outcry spurred by Adams's *Great American Fraud* and Upton Sinclair's novel about the unsanitary business of meat packing, *The Jungle* (1906), the federal government passed the Food and Drug Act, which established the Food and Drug Administration (FDA) to, among other thing, keep dangerous and fraudulent medicines in check. Although loopholes in the original law prevented the FDA from initially wielding much power against the pharmaceutical industry, the agency provided legitimacy for the AMA's continued mission to curb the influence of patent medicines, and a 1912 amendment to the act began to prohibit fraudulent claims of effectiveness made by advertisements for proprietary medicine. This further limited the ability of marketers to mention a specific diagnosis such as neurasthenia, because to do so carried the responsibility to actually cure the illness. Beginning in 1913, state legislatures assisted in the attempt to clamp down on medical advertising by passing an advertising law known as The Model Statute, which made it a misdemeanor for an "advertisement of any sort" to make "any assertion, representation or statement of fact which is untrue, deceptive or misleading." By 1922, twenty-three states had passed the statute and Better Business Bureaus around the nation were spearheading a truth-in-advertising movement that placed further pressure on media sources to refrain from publishing the types of advertisements that a generation before were popularizing neurasthenia (as well as yielding pharmaceutical companies massive profits).[29]

Succumbing to pressure from the AMA, muckraking journalists, the courts, and government legislatures, by 1920 patent medicine companies severely curbed their volume of advertisements that tried to convince people that they were sick with neurasthenia. The strategy to get Americans to self-diagnosis and self-medicate was lucrative, but it also attracted accusations of fraud and recklessness that eventually forced companies to modify their advertising by retreating from "cure-all" claims and specific medical diagnoses.[30]

Miles Medical Company remained a successful business, eventually changing its name to Miles Laboratories and diversifying its product line with the development of Alka-Seltzer (1931), One-A-Day (1940) and Flintstone (1969) vitamins, Bactine antiseptic (1950), and the Morningstar Farms line of cholesterol-free meat substitutes (1973), before merging with the West German pharmaceutical giant Bayer in 1979. Miles Medical continued to market Nervine well after the 1920s, using much of the same language and explanations for health that it did in the late nineteenth century but with illnesses only alluded to rather than specifically mentioned. "Modern living conditions with their noise, excitement, worry, confining work, [and] fear of the future use up our Nerve Force more rapidly than Nature can replace it," a Nervine ad from Dr. Miles's 1936 almanac read; "Restlessness, Irritability, Sleeplessness are early signs of an over-taxed nervous system, [and] that jumping Headache or that attack of Indigestion may be due to 'NERVES.' "[31] Nervine ads continued to utilize the theory of nervous energy that once helped define neurasthenia, but they no longer mentioned either neurasthenia or its cognates, nervous exhaustion or nervous prostration. In this way the idea behind neurasthenia—that health, happiness, and comfort were intertwined—continued to be part of America's therapeutic language but the diagnosis of neurasthenia did not.

The neurasthenia diagnosis fell out of use in the twentieth century because of changes within the American medical profession. What were once strengths of the diagnosis—its protean nature, its easily applicable concept of nervous energy, patient affinity—were out of step with the more tightly regulated profession that the American Medical Association built after its 1901 reorganization. Whereas doctors insisted on more diagnostic specificity, neurasthenia was vague. Whereas physicians demanded scientific evidence to back up etiologies, nervous energy was unproven. Whereas the medical profession sought to become the definitive opinion source on medical issues, neurasthenia was popularized. Newly discovered hormones and vitamins chipped away at the neurasthenia diagnosis by displacing nervous energy as the source of good health. Most important from a medical perspective, though, leaders in neurology, the specialty built upon neurasthenia, recognized that their discipline had fallen behind their erstwhile competitors' in psychiatry and began the move to recast neurasthenic symptoms as more rigorously defined psychiatric and psychological conditions. The AMA's campaign to regulate patent medicines and discourage self-diagnosis and self-treatment also contributed to the decline of neurasthenia, by helping to take specific mention of the condition out of advertising. Thus, at approximately the same time, both the medical profession and the pharmaceutical industry were reducing their reliance on the diagnosis to further their industries.

By 1920 the newest generation of Americans understood neurasthenia as a dated disease from which their parents and grandparents suffered. In that year, the census showed that cities, once a novelty that reportedly drained Americans of their energy, had become the norm and home to more Americans than rural areas. The proliferation of downtown skyscrapers signaled that office jobs, once feared as the source of sedentary brain work, had become the active center of an energetic American economy. The "dollar devil" that supposedly tempted people to overwork themselves into sickness had been balanced by department stores, new cathedrals of consumption that sold products that promised happiness and comfort. Women's suffrage in 1920 resolved a social issue that had been brewing for over seventy years, and lowered the volume of debate over the role of women, until its rising once more in the 1960s. The popular appeal of Warren G. Harding's election promise of a "return to normalcy" demonstrates that, by 1920, people were ready to look idyllically at the past as a time of rest and calm rather than of fatigue and anxiety.

Epilogue

Neurasthenia's Legacy

On September 5, 2004, the *New York Times* ran a front-page feature titled "Always at Work and Anxious: Employees' Health Is Suffering." The paper reported that 53 percent of American workers claimed that their jobs left them "overtired and overwhelmed," a stressful combination researchers had linked to heart disease, stroke, diabetes, and weakened immune systems. Downsizing, outsourcing, economic insecurity, capricious management, and pressure to raise productivity have made people feel powerless at work, while technological gadgets such as cell phones and laptops have made it impossible for people to relax away from their jobs. Quoting a physician, the *Times* posited that humans were not made "to handle the chronic stress that is an inescapable accompaniment of modern life. The wear and tear of long hours, ringing phones, uncertain work conditions, and family demands" caused "fatigue, frustration, anger, and burnout." This was reportedly a new phenomenon that researchers were just now "beginning to document."[1]

On one level, this news story appears to be a case of social amnesia in which America's past experience with neurasthenia has been completely forgotten, yet it also demonstrates how thoroughly America still feels neurasthenia's influence in the twenty-first century. The United States has long wrestled with the question Beard raised with the diagnosis back in 1869: how can Americans stay healthy while struggling with the demands of modern life? Every generation has developed its own way of speaking of health that encapsulates much of what neurasthenia stood for.[2] The reciprocal cycle of information has remained part of this process, as it has continued to make the language of health reflective at the same time of developments in professional medicine,

of the personal experience of patients, and of popular culture. Americans'
search for health, happiness, and comfort became one of the defining themes in
twentieth-century plays and novels; the idea of *nervous breakdown* quickly
picked up where the public's understanding of neurasthenia left off; the concept
of stress essentially became a twentieth-century parallel to the idea of lacking
nervous energy; the "problem that had no name" became an incarnation of
housewives' neurasthenia; and, by the turn of the twenty-first century, scholars
were hailing a new generation of chronic illnesses as the progeny of neurasthenia.

The relationship that neurasthenia highlighted between health and
lifestyle served as an influential theme in twentieth-century American literature. George S. Kaufman and Moss Hart's comedy *You Can't Take It With You*
(1936), for instance, relied on a contrast between two diametrically opposed
families, the free-spirited Vanderhofs and the serious-minded Kirbys. The
Vanderhof household was in constant chaos as each member followed his or
her individual interests, be these ballet, making fireworks, or playing the xylo-
phone, in a manner reminiscent of George M. Beard's suggestion that people
needed to worry less and play more. Confusion abounded, but so did health,
happiness, and comfort. The Kirbys were tightly wound, by comparison, and
Mr. Kirby, a successful businessman, was perpetually upset and suffered from
chronic indigestion. In the final act, Grandpa Vanderhof explained to Mr. Kirby
the key to health that the neurasthenia diagnosis had established more than
sixty-five years earlier. "What do you think you get your indigestion from?"
Grandpa asked Mr. Kirby; "Happiness? No, sir. You get it because most of your
time is spent in doing things you don't want to do." Grandpa explained how he
used to worry himself sick over work and politics, but decided to give it all up
and has been happy and healthy ever since. The advice had a miraculous effect
on Mr. Kirby, who quickly embraced Grandpa's carefree attitude and found
at the end of the play that his indigestion had disappeared.[3] The play does not
specifically mention *neurasthenia*, but the tension between health and work
that the diagnosis helped illuminate a generation before is unmistakable.

The dynamic between health and modern life found in neurasthenia also
served as the backdrop of Saul Bellow's *Seize the Day* (1956). Protagonist
Tommy Wilhelm had many opportunities in life, but success and happiness
always seemed just out of reach. His career as an actor, his marriage, his relationship with his sons, and his relationship with his father all disintegrated for
reasons that he felt were beyond his control. The result was "so much bad luck,
weariness, weakness, and failure." As did neurasthenics, Wilhelm craved for
someone to "care about him, wish him well. Kindness, mercy, he wanted." His
father, a famous surgeon, offered little help, preferring to keep his "sympathy

for real ailments" and to criticize his son for "indulging himself too much in his emotions." Wilhelm was a tragic figure whose decisions kept having painful outcomes; as neurasthenics often did, he relied on the regular use of medication as a "boost against . . . misery," and, in a desperate attempt to redeem himself financially, entered into a business partnership in which he lost the remainder of his savings on the stock market. "You've got to keep your nerve when the market starts to go places," his shady partner lectured him; "This is the difference between healthiness and pathology." An emotional wreck whose life had collapsed around him, at the end of the book Wilhelm breaks down and cries uncontrollably at the funeral of a person he never knew. Bellow's story was essentially a psychological profile of a man having a neurasthenic breakdown, unable to withstand the burdens of supporting his estranged family, being alienated from his father, and losing money in the dog-eat-dog capitalist system.[4]

During the mid-1950s Americans would have identified Wilhelm as suffering from a nervous breakdown rather than from neurasthenia. The term *nervous breakdown* became part of the popular consciousness after 1901 as the title of a short volume by San Francisco physician Albert Abrams. Abrams described the condition as the noxious product of neurasthenia that robbed people of "their enjoyments of pleasure and the comforts of life." Nervous breakdown symptoms remained consistent with typical descriptions of neurasthenia and included insomnia, depression, irrationality, sexual dysfunction, fatigue, indigestion, and constipation. Abrams's *Nervous Breakdown* provided Americans with a dramatic way of speaking of neurasthenia that quickly caught on but always remained an informal concept, generally avoided by physicians for being too vague—it was originally associated with neurasthenia, after all. The vague nature of *nervous breakdown* made it a favorite informal diagnosis among the lay public, who continued to use it into the second half of the twentieth century to describe their personal health, well after the neurasthenia diagnosis had faded into memory. An important distinction between the neurasthenia and nervous breakdown descriptors is that, whereas people understood neurasthenia as a grinding chronic illness that caused discomfort and impinged on happiness, a nervous breakdown came to represent the snapping point when discomfort and unhappiness became unbearable.[5]

Although doctors tried to avoid the language of nervous breakdown, the larger American public widely embraced the concept as the heir to neurasthenia. Since *nervous breakdown* was only an informal term, drug companies had freer rein to refer to the condition in their advertising without provoking a regulatory response. As a result, products such as Nervine went from being marketed as cures for neurasthenia to being sold to cure nervous breakdowns. "I had a nervous breakdown and was in very bad condition," a 1936 Miles Medical testimonial read; "I have now taken twelve bottles of Nervine and am feeling fine." Popular health handbooks like Abrams's and advertisements for medicines were only a few of the sources that trained Americans in the linguistic transition between neurasthenia and nervous breakdown. The popular press wove nervous breakdowns into stories just as it had previously done with neurasthenia during the late nineteenth and early twentieth centuries. F. Scott Fitzgerald wrote a series of three introspective articles for *Esquire* in 1936 documenting his own nervous breakdown, later published as the compilation *The Crack-up*. In 1956 the *Saturday Evening Post* even credited Walt Disney's whimsical nature to a nervous breakdown he suffered after being betrayed by a fellow animator: the breakdown taught him not to take work so seriously, "so he decided to have fun, just like his own creations."[6] As a condition of the artistic and successful, nervous breakdowns carried much of neurasthenia's fashionable aura.

In a progression accelerating after 1920, journalists, writers, and advertisers essentially began swapping out references to neurasthenia for references to nervous breakdowns. A comparison between how often stories and advertisements in the *New York Times* mentioned *neurasthenia* and its cognates (*nervous prostration* and *nervous exhaustion*) with how often it mentioned *nervous breakdown*, *psychosis*, and *neurosis* reveals that during the very years that neurasthenia was fading from public view within the pages of the newspaper, the ideas of psychosis, neurosis, and—above all—nervous breakdown were on the rise to take neurasthenia's place. During neurasthenia's heyday, from 1890 to 1899, the *Times* mentioned it and its cognates 875 times compared with merely 33 references to nervous breakdowns, psychoses, and neuroses. The next decade saw references to neurasthenia increase slightly to 900, but the shift toward speaking of nervous breakdown, neuroses, and psychoses is evident with 225 references. From 1910 to 1919, the linguistic handoff between neurasthenia and nervous breakdowns, neuroses, and psychoses was well underway, with mention of neurasthenia falling to 546 and the others increasing to 626. During the decade of the 1920s, the *Times* only mentioned neurasthenia 248 times, a drop of nearly 55 percent from the previous decade, while references to nervous breakdowns, neuroses, and psychoses increased over 70 percent, to 1071.[7] Inasmuch as the *Times* is an indicator of conversations going on in America, people were talking about their health, happiness, and comfort more than ever after 1920; they were just leaving neurasthenia out of the discussion.

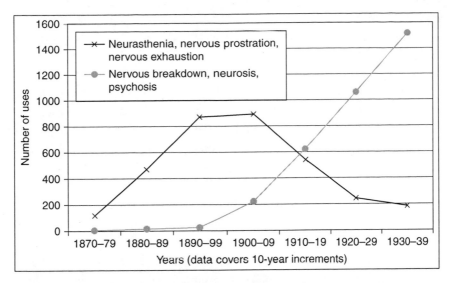

Data (number of times each term was used by the *New York Times* during a particular decade)

				Decades				
Term:	(1870–1930 total)	1870–79	1880–89	1890–99	1900–09	1910–19	1920–29	1930 39
Nervous prostration:	2,173	117	399	762	582	195	79	39
Nervous exhaustion:	447	7	63	83	77	74	63	80
Neurasthenia:	735	0	9	30	241	277	106	72
Nervous breakdown:	2,320	0	1	1	179	495	775	869
Neurosis:	656	11	18	28	31	80	165	323
Psychosis:	533	0	2	4	15	51	131	330
NP + NE + N	3,355	124	471	875	900	546	248	191
NB + Nr + Ps	3,509	11	21	33	225	626	1,071	1,522

Figure 14 Graph of *New York Times* references to neurasthenic conditions. As the *Times* decreased mention of neurasthenia and its related diagnoses (nervous prostration and nervous exhaustion), it began increasing mention of neuroses, psychoses, and nervous breakdowns, all conditions that displaced neurasthenia within America's medical and popular lexicon.

While the mid twentieth-century public spoke of nervous breakdowns, endocrinologist Hans Selye's research on stress began to transform the way physicians and laypeople alike understood the impact of day-to-day life on health. Beginning with a short article published in *Nature* in 1936 and culminating in his widely read *The Stress of Life* (1956), Selye extended the research done on hormones during the first part of the century to identify what he hoped would become a "unified theory of disease." Much as Mitchell introduced Americans to the concept of neurasthenia in 1871, Selye announced that "stress is essentially the rate of all the wear and tear caused by life"; "The secret of health and happiness," he claimed, "lies in successful adjustment to the ever-changing conditions on this globe." The interplay among people, their surroundings, and their health represented what Selye called the *general adaptation syndrome* (GAS), in which the body's endocrine glands and nervous system sought to adjust to constant physical, psychological, and emotional changes. "The penalties for failure in this great process of adaptation are disease and unhappiness," Selye explained in the preface to *The Stress of Life*.[8] Stress, like nervous energy before it, helped explain a wide variety of otherwise unexplainable symptoms, but, unlike the unproven concept of nervous energy, the concept of stress could be traced to specific hormonal and physiological processes, thereby securing its place in twentieth-century scientific medicine as well as in the popular imagination.

The interplay between health and gender roles, especially female domesticity, that was part of the dialogue surrounding neurasthenia continued in different guises into the second part of the twentieth century. In the first published article on neurasthenia in 1869, E. H. Van Deusen remarked how young farm wives often fell sick with neurasthenia because of the despair they experienced after leaving their family and friends to live on an isolated farm with their new husbands, and Charlotte Perkins Gilman had written a handful of articles linking neurasthenia to restrictive gender roles. In 1920, Abraham Myerson published *The Nervous Housewife*, which reiterated many of Gilman's calls for allowing women to modernize their domestic responsibilities for the sake of personal health. As neurasthenia faded from public and professional discourse, so did the links between domesticity, discomfort, and unhappiness, until Betty Friedan picked up the issue in *The Feminine Mystique* (1963). In what she called the "problem that has no name," Friedan linked many of the physical and psychological ailments suffered by American women after the Second World War to an American culture and society that defined women's responsibilities as purely domestic. She compiled examples of the psychological and physical effects of domesticity, including constant fatigue, irritability, unexplained sores, hopelessness, the overwhelming need to cry—all symptoms given nicknames such as "housewife's syndrome," "housewife's blight," and "housewife's fatigue" and treated by the medical profession with tranquilizers and psychotherapy. A 1972 abnormal psychology textbook called the domestic sickness "housewives' neurosis" and connected it explicitly to the antiquated neurasthenia diagnosis and "housewives who are bored and feel neglected by their husbands." Such a definition most likely would have rankled both Friedan and Gilman because it lodged responsibility for sickness with women themselves rather than in the unhealthy consequences of domesticity.[9]

It is difficult to ignore shadows of neurasthenia in the late-twentieth-century proliferation of chronic illness diagnoses. Scholars have argued that chronic fatigue syndrome, bipolar disorder, fibromyalgia, post-traumatic stress disorder, irritable bowel syndrome, myalgic encephalomyelitis (ME), mononucleosis, environmental allergies, and a host of anxiety and depressive disorders are all modern equivalents of neurasthenia. Aside from their chronic nature and tendency for the afflicted to have good and bad days, what these diagnoses all share with neurasthenia is their ability to recognize unhappiness and discomfort despite the lack of an obvious—especially by late-nineteenth-century standards—organic cause. They also connect emotional health to physical well-being by making depression and irritability a common accompaniment to physical symptoms. As with neurasthenia, these conditions often prompted people to adopt lifestyle changes, such as increasing exercise, changing diet, and avoiding overwork and anxiety, in hope of improving overall health. Finally, some of these diagnoses of chronic conditions have come under criticism, as neurasthenia did, from those inside and outside the medical profession as "waste bin" diagnoses, too vague and generalized to meet the rigorous diagnostic standards of scientific medicine.[10]

Marginalized by the medical profession and displaced in the public mind by other conditions after 1920, neurasthenia was eventually eliminated altogether as an official diagnosis by the American Psychiatric Association in the 1980 edition of its *Diagnostic Statistical Manual* (DSM III). Although there was a push by some advocates to get neurasthenia reinstated as a diagnosis in the DSM IV, practitioners within the United States were content to leave neurasthenia part of their nation's medical history. Ironically, the diagnosis once celebrated as the "American disease" is still commonly used elsewhere in the world, including China (where it corresponds well with traditional Chinese concepts of medicine) and countries previously associated with the Soviet bloc. The United Nations' World Health Organization also recognizes neurasthenia as a legitimate disease in its most recent *International Classification of Diseases* (ICD-10) and given the condition's protean and easily applicable nature, it will most likely remain an active part of the medical lexicon outside the United States for a long time to come.[11]

Within the United States, habits that the concept of neurasthenia helped cultivate continue to influence the way Americans approach health care. Like patent medicine companies in the past, pharmaceutical manufacturers are today spending impressive sums of money to advertise their products directly to consumers (still to the chagrin of many within the medical profession) in hope of getting Americans to self-diagnose and seek a drug treatment. A 2008 survey found that nearly half of all American physicians have relied on placebo prescriptions to combat the emotional and physical symptoms of chronic illness, a therapeutic approach akin to Beard's electrotherapy and the power of suggestion that many physicians relied on to treat neurasthenia. Another study found that, between 1997 and 2005, sales of the nation's top five painkillers increased by 90 percent, an indication that Americans are again seeking relief from life's discomforts in a bottle, as they once did with patent medicines. The pernicious impact of modern life on the mental health of Americans convinced a number of psychologists at the start of the twenty-first century that the time had come to join forces with the nation's clergy to create an alliance of counseling services, an endeavor that echoes the goal of the Emmanuel Movement a century earlier.[12] The word *neurasthenia* may not be readily recognized by Americans today, but the search for health, happiness, and comfort that grew out of people's struggle with the illness represents its lasting legacy.

Notes

The following archival holdings have provided the grist for much of this book's research. After each holding is the shortened reference used in the notes.

George M. Beard Papers, Manuscripts and Archives, Yale University Library (Beard Papers).

Mitchell Papers, College of Physicians of Philadelphia (CPP).

Advertising Ephemera Collection, John W. Hartman Center for Sales, Advertising and Marketing History, Rare Book, Manuscript, and Special Collections Library, Duke University (Hartman Center).

Nervous disease cases, Cooper Medical College records, Special Collections, Lane Medical Library, Stanford University (CMC).

S. Weir Mitchell Papers, History of Medicine Collection, Medical Center Library, Duke University (MP-DML).

James Jackson Putnam Papers, Center for the History of Medicine, Francis A. Countway Library of Medicine (JJPP-CLM).

Frederick Cheever Shattuck Papers, Center for the History of Medicine, Francis A. Countway Library of Medicine (FCS-CLM).

Bancroft Library, University of California, Berkeley (Bancroft Library).

Introduction

1. G. Alder Blumer, "The Coming of Psychesthenia," *Journal of Nervous and Mental Diseases* 33 (1906): 336.

2. Donna B. Greenberg, "Neurasthenia in the 1980s: Chronic Mononucleosis, Chronic Fatigue Syndrome, and Anxiety and Depressive Disorders," *Psychosomatics* 31 (Spring 1990): 129–137; Susan E. Abby and Paul E. Garfinkel, "Neurasthenia and Chronic Fatigue Syndrome: The Role of Culture in the Making of a Diagnosis," *American Journal of Psychiatry* 148 (December 1991): 1638–1646; Edward Shorter, "Chronic Fatigue in Historical Perspective," *Ciba Foundation Symposium* 173 (1993): 6–22.

3. Marijke Gijswijt-Hofstra and Roy Porter, eds., *Cultures of Neurasthenia: From Beard to the First World War* (New York: Rodopi, 2001); Arthur Kleinman, *Social Origins of Distress and Disease: Depression, Neurasthenia, and Pain in Modern China* (New Haven, Conn.: Yale University Press, 1986).

4. Morton Prince, "Hysterical Neurasthenia," *Boston Medical and Surgical Journal* 139 (December 29, 1898): 652–655; J. T. Eskridge, "Some Points in the Diagnosis of Traumatic Injuries of the Central Nervous System," *Journal of the American Medical Association* 34 (March 10, 1900): 579–584; "Traumatic Hysteria: Discussion on Dr. Booth's Paper in March Issue," *International Journal of Surgery* 19 (May 1906): 181–182; Ernst S. Reynolds, "Hysteria and Neurasthenia," *British Medical Journal* 2 (December 22, 1923): 1193–1196; S. Weir Mitchell, *Fat and Blood: An Essay on the Treatment of Certain Forms of Neurasthenia and Hysteria*, 3d ed. (Philadelphia: J. B. Lippincott and Co., 1884).

5. Elaine Showalter, *The Female Malady: Women, Madness, and English Culture, 1830–1980* (New York: Penguin Books, 1985); Janet Oppenheim, *"Shattered Nerves": Doctors, Patients, and Depression in Victorian England* (New York: Oxford University Press, 1991); Mark S. Micale, *Hysterical Men: The Hidden History of Male Nervous Illness* (Cambridge, Mass.: Harvard University Press, 2008); Andrew Scull, *Hysteria: The Biography* (New York: Oxford University Press, 2009).

Chapter 1 — Professional Medicine and the Discovery of Neurasthenia

1. James J. Putnam, "Remarks on the Psychical Treatment of Neurasthenia," *Boston Medical and Surgical Journal* 132 (May 23, 1895): 505; Charles L. Dana, "The Partial Passing of Neurasthenia," *Boston Medical and Surgical Journal* 150 (March 31, 1904): 341.

2. The term *neurasthenia* was not entirely original, and Van Deusen and Beard each acknowledged that he co-opted the phrase *nervous asthenia* from a brief description found in an earlier medical text by Austin Flint. See Flint, *A Treatise on the Principles and Practice of Medicine; Designed for the Use of Practitioners and Students of Medicine* (Philadelphia: Henry C. Lea, 1866), 640–641. "Neurasthenia" could also be found as a short entry in Robley Dunglison's *Dictionary of Medical Science* (Philadelphia: Lea and Blanchard, 1846).

3. Barbara Sicherman recognized the reciprocity created by neurasthenia between patients and physicians in "The Uses of a Diagnosis: Doctors, Patients, and Neurasthenia," in *Sickness and Health in America*, Judith Walzer Leavitt and Ronald L. Numbers, eds. (Madison: University of Wisconsin Press, 1985), 22–35. Andrew Abbott also used the doctor-patient relationship created by neurasthenia as a case study in *The System of Professions: An Essay on the Division of Expert Labor* (Chicago: University of Chicago Press, 1988), 280–314.

4. "Dr. E. H. Van Deusen Is Dead after Long Illness," *Kalamazoo Gazette*, July 10, 1909.

5. For biographical information on Van Deusen, see his obituaries in the *Kalamazoo Gazette*, July 10, 1909, and the *Report of the Board of Trustees of the Michigan Asylum for the Insane* (Lansing: Wynkoop Hallenbeck Crawford Co., 1910), 15–16; name entry in *Cyclopedia of Michigan; Historical and Biographical* (New York: Western Pub. and Engraving Co., 1890), 307–308; David Fisher, "Dr. E. H. Van Deusen," *Compendium of History and Biography of Kalamazoo County, Michigan* (Chicago: A. W. Bowen and Co., 1906), 117–118; John M. McCormick, "Dr. Edwin Holmes Van Deusen," *Historical Collections of the Michigan Pioneer and Historical Society* 38 (Lansing: Michigan Pioneer and Historical Society, 1912), 728–731; Albert Grady, "The Life of Dr. Edwin Van Deusen (1828–1910)" (unpublished papers from the History Seminar of Kalamazoo College, January 1949). These sources can be found in the Edwin H. Van Deusen name file at the Kalamazoo Public Library, Local History Room.

6. Grady, "The Life of Dr. Edwin Van Deusen," 12; E. H. Van Deusen, "Observations on a Form of Nervous Prostration, (Neurasthenia,) Culminating in Insanity," *American Journal of Insanity* 15 (April 1869): 447. Van Deusen actually wrote his article on neurasthenia a few years earlier for inclusion in his report to trustees; see "Observations on a Form of Nervous Prostration, (Neurasthenia,) Culminating in Insanity," *Supplement to the Report of the Board of Trustees for the Michigan Asylum for the Insane, 1867–68* (Lansing: W. S. George and Co.: Printers of the State, 1869), 3–19. Future quotations from Van Deusen's article use the *American Journal of Insanity* pagination.

7. Van Deusen, "Observations on a Form of Nervous Prostration," 446–447, 457.

8. Ibid., 445–446, 450–451.

9. Ibid., 454–455, 457, 461. For more on moral treatment found in nineteenth century American asylums, see Nancy Tomes, *The Art of Asylum Keeping: Thomas Story Kirkbride and the Origins of American Psychiatry* (Philadelphia: University of Pennsylvania Press, 1994).

10. David J. Rothman, *The Discovery of the Asylum: Social Order and Disorder in the New Republic* (Boston: Scott, Foresman and Co., 1971), 131; Gerald Grob, *Mental Institutions in American Society: Social Policy to 1875* (New York: Free Press, 1973); Grob, *Mental Illness and American Society, 1875–1940* (Princeton: Princeton University Press, 1983); Tomes, *Art of Asylum Keeping*; Lynn Gamwell and Nancy Tomes, *Madness in America: Cultural and Medical Perceptions of Mental Illness before 1914* (Ithaca, N.Y.: Cornell University Press, 1995), 55.

11. Edgar Allen Poe, "The System of Dr. Tarr and Prof. Fether," *Graham's Magazine* 28 (November 1845): 193–200; Isaac Hunt, *Three Years in a Mad-House* (Skowhegan, Maine: A. A. Mann, 1851); Ebenezer Haskell, *The Trial of Ebenezer Haskell, in Lunacy . . .* (Philadelphia: E. Haskell, 1869); Nellie Bly, *Ten Days in a Mad-House* (New York: Ian L. Munro, 1887). Gamwell and Tomes give a useful account of anti-asylum literature in *Madness in America*, 63–65, 122–124.

12. *Van Deusen v. Newcomer*, 40 Mich. 90 (Mich. 1879).

13. *Ibid.*; Fischer, "Dr. E. H. Van Deusen," 118. Grob mentions the Newcomer case, although not specifically by name, in *Mental Illness in American Society*, 49–50.

14. Charles E. Rosenberg, *The Trial of the Assassin Guiteau: Psychiatry and Law in the Gilded Age* (Chicago: University of Chicago Press, 1968), 71–74; Grob, *Mental Illness in American Society*, 49–55; F. G. Gosling, *Before Freud: Neurasthenia and the American Medical Community, 1870–1910* (Chicago: University of Illinois Press, 1987), 19–21; Rothman, *Discovery of the Asylum*, 268–269.

15. George M. Beard, *The Psychology of the Salem Witchcraft Excitement of 1692 and Its Practical Application to Our Own Time* (New York: G. P. Putnam's Sons, 1882), xvii–xviii.

16. Janet Oppenheim also made the rural-urban distinction between Van Deusen and neurologists such as Beard and Mitchell in *"Shattered Nerves": Doctors, Patients, and Depression in Victorian England* (New York: Oxford University Press, 1991), 92–93. Charles Rosenberg, "The Place of George M. Beard in Nineteenth-Century Psychiatry," *Bulletin of the History of Medicine* 36 (May–June 1962): 245–259.

17. George M. Beard, "Neurasthenia, or Nervous Exhaustion," *Boston Medical and Surgical Journal* 3 (April 29, 1869): 217–221; George M. Beard, *A Practical Treatise on Nervous Exhaustion (Neurasthenia)* (New York: W. Wood and Co., 1880); George M. Beard, *American Nervousness: Its Causes and Consequences* (New York: G. P. Putnam's Sons, 1881). For a convenient list of most of Beard's many publications, see Philip P. Wiener, "G. M. Beard and Freud on 'American Nervousness,'" *Journal of the History of Ideas* 17 (April 1956): 269–274.

18. Much of the biographical information about Beard comes from Roger S. Tracy, "George Miller Beard," *Twenty Years' Record*, 1, 7–8 (Yale University Alumni publication, circa 1883) found in the Beard Papers, box 3, folder 7. Other useful sources of information about Beard include Rosenberg's "The Place of George M. Beard" and Charles L. Dana's "Dr. George M. Beard: A Sketch of His Life and Character, with Some Personal Reminiscences," *Archive of Neurology and Psychiatry* 10 (1923): 427–435.

19. Gosling, *Before Freud*, 20–22; Rosenberg, "The Place of George M. Beard," 249; Oppenheim, *"Shattered Nerves,"* 79–109.

20. Tracy, "George Miller Beard," 1. Works co-authored by Beard and Rockwell include: *The Medical Use of Electricity, with Special Reference to General Electrization* (New York: William Wood, 1867); *Observations on the Physiological and Therapeutical Effects of Galvanization of the Sympathetic* (New York: New York Publishing Co., 1870); and *A Practical Treatise on the Medical and Surgical Uses of Electricity* (New York: W. Wood and Co., 1871).

21. Tracy, "George Miller Beard," 3, 7–8; Beard, "The Psychology of Spiritualism," *The North American Review* 129 (July 1879): 65–80; Thomas Edison to Grace A. Beard, October 15, 1908, Beard Papers, box 1, folder 18; Beard, "The Nature of the Newly Discovered Force," *Scientific American* 34 (January 22, 1876): 57; Beard, "Longevity of Brain-Workers," *Hours at Home* 5 (1867): 511–517; Beard, "Popular Fallacies Concerning Hygiene, part 2: Fallacies Relating to Hereditary Genius," *Appletons' Journal of Literature, Science, and Art* 20 (August 14, 1869): 625–627.

22. John C. Burnham, *How Superstition Won and Science Lost: Popularizing Science and Health in the United States* (New Brunswick, N.J.: Rutgers University Press, 1987), 21–44; John Harley Warner, *The Therapeutic Perspective: Medical Practice, Knowledge, and Identity in America, 1820–1885* (Cambridge, Mass.: Harvard University Press, 1986), 223; Beard, "Popular Fallacies Concerning Hygiene, part 2," 625; Beard, *American Nervousness*, vi. For an example of Beard's faith in the power of experts to recognize the truth, see the preface to his *Psychology of the Salem Witchcraft Excitement*, v–xx.

23. R. Laurence Moore, *In Search of White Crows: Spiritualism, Parapsychology, and American Culture* (New York: Oxford University Press, 1977), 3; Stephen R. Prothero, *The White Buddhist: The Asian Odyssey of Henry Steel Olcott* (Bloomington: Indiana University Press, 1996).

24. Henry S. Olcott, *People from the Other World* (Hartford, Conn.: American Publishing Company, 1875).

25. George M. Beard, "The Eddy Mediums," *The Daily Graphic*, November 9, 1874, 57–58; "Spiritual Manifestations of the Eddy Brothers," *Medical and Surgical Reporter* 32 (January 2, 1875): 17. The "benumbing arm trick" that Beard referred to was this: with cold hands and under cover of a blanket, the spiritualist would grasp the arm of a participant with both hands so that the participant could feel the grasp but not see it. Then, gently, the spiritualist would release the grip of his lower hand, thereby freeing it to play instruments or otherwise create the illusion that a spiritual force was at work. If the grip of the spiritualist's upper hand was firm enough, the participant would not notice that the lower grip was loosened and, because of the blanket, he or she would not see this either.

26. Beard, *American Nervousness*, 96.

27. Ibid., 101–112; Beard, "Neurasthenia, or Nervous Exhaustion," 217–218.

28. Beard, *American Nervousness*, 117, 121, 128–131.

29. Ibid., viii; George M. Beard, *Herbert Spencer on American Nervousness: A Scientific Coincidence* (New York: G. P. Putnam's Sons, 1883), 12.

30. Beard, *American Nervousness*, 126, 130–132, 181–192.

31. Ibid., xvii, vii–viii.

32. Mary O. Furner, *Advocacy and Objectivity: A Crisis in the Professionalization of American Social Science, 1865–1905* (Lexington: University Press of Kentucky, 1975); Thomas Haskell, *The Emergence of Professional Social Science: The*

American Social Science Association and the Nineteenth-Century Crisis of Authority (Urbana: University of Illinois Press, 1977); Dorothy Ross, *The Origins of American Social Science* (New York: Cambridge University Press, 1991).

33. George M. Beard, "The Influence of the Mind in the Causation and Cure of Disease—The Potency of Definite Expectation," *Journal of Nervous and Mental Disease* 3 (1876): 429–437; Beard, "Mental Therapeutics," *Journal of Nervous and Mental Disease* 4 (1877): 581–582. The story of Beard and his dead battery came from neurologist Charles Dana who, as a young physician, worked with Beard (see Dana, "Dr. George M. Beard"). Gosling discusses the efficacy of various neurasthenia treatments in *Before Freud*, 108–142. Henry K. Beecher, "The Powerful Placebo," *Journal of the American Medical Association* 159 (December 24, 1955): 1602–1606.

34. George M. Beard, "Recent Works on the Brain and Nerves," *North American Review* 131 (September 1880): 284.

35. Roberts Bartholow, "What Is Meant by Nervous Prostration?" *Medical and Surgical Reporter* 50 (January 26, 1884): 97.

36. "The Cause of Dr. Beard's Death," *New York Times*, January 25, 1883, 3.

37. For biographical information on Mitchell, see Ernest Earnest, *S. Weir Mitchell: Novelist and Physician* (Philadelphia: University of Pennsylvania Press, 1950); Anna Robeson Burr, ed., *Weir Mitchell: His Life and Letters* (New York: Duffield and Co., 1929), 140; Frederick P. Henry, "Tribute to S. Weir Mitchell," in *S. Weir Mitchell: Memorial Addresses and Resolutions* (Philadelphia: College of Physicians of Philadelphia, 1914), 39–40; Lawrence C. McHenry, *Garrison's History of Neurology* (Springfield, Ill.: Charles C. Thomas, 1969), 327.

38. S. Weir Mitchell, *Researches upon Venom of the Rattlesnake, with Investigation of Anatomy and Physiology of the Organs Concerned*, Smithsonian Contributions to Knowledge series, vol. 12, art. 6 (Washington, D.C.: Smithsonian Institute, 1860); S. Weir Mitchell, George R. Morehouse, and William W. Keen, *Gunshot Wounds and Other Injuries of Nerves* (Philadelphia: J. B. Lippincott, 1864); S. Weir Mitchell, George R. Morehouse, William W. Keen, and John F. Fulton, *Reflex Paralysis: A Reprint with Introduction* (New Haven, Conn.: Historical Library, Yale University School of Medicine, 1941; reprinted from Surgeon General's Office, Circular no. 6, March 10, 1864; new introduction by John F. Fulton).

39. S. Weir Mitchell, *Doctor and Patient* (Philadelphia: J.B. Lippincott, 1888), 10.

40. Amelia Gere Mason to S. Weir Mitchell, February 17, 1912; Mason to John K. Mitchell, November 30, 1914: CPP series 4.3, box 9. All other correspondence between Mason and Mitchell comes from the same series and box.

41. Mason to Mitchell, December 27, 1886, CPP; Mason to Mitchell, February 10, 1911, CPP.

42. Mitchell, *Doctor and Patient*, 88, 155–157, 173; Suzanne Poirier, "The Weir Mitchell Rest Cure: Doctors and Patients," *Women's Studies* 10 (January 1983): 15–40; Mitchell, *Nurse and Patient, and Camp Cure* (Philadelphia: J. B. Lippincott, 1877). Edmund Wilson forwarded the idea that Mitchell encouraged Edith Wharton to start writing, a claim that other scholars have questioned. See Wilson, *The Wound and the Bow: Seven Studies in Literature* (London: University Paperbacks, 1961), 175. For opposition to Wilson's claim, see Grace Kellogg, *The Two Lives of Edith Wharton: The Woman and Her Work* (New York: Appleton-Century, 1965), 84; and Olivia Coolidge, *Edith Wharton* (New York: Scribner, 1964), 66.

43. S. Weir Mitchell, *Fat and Blood and How to Make Them*, 2nd ed. (Philadelphia: J. B. Lippincott, 1878), 9; Joan Jacob Brumberg, *Fasting Girls: The Emergence of Anorexia*

Nervosa as a Modern Disease (Cambridge, Mass.: Harvard University Press, 1988), 141–163; Oppenheim, *"Shattered Nerves,"* 211–216.

44. Mitchell, *Fat and Blood*, 73–106.

45. Ibid., 41–42; R. B., Review of *Fat and Blood and How to Make Them*, by S. Weir Mitchell, *The American Journal of the Medical Sciences* 75 (January 1878): 198.

46. For historical studies on the importance of authority and trust in the treatment of neurasthenia, see Gosling, 62–63; and Sicherman, "The Uses of a Diagnosis: Doctors, Patients, and Neurasthenia," 22–35. Mitchell, *Fat and Blood*, 41; Mitchell, *Doctor and Patient*, 125, 11; Mason to Mitchell, July 7, 1892, CPP.

47. E. L. Dana to S. Weir Mitchell, March 9, 1902, box 10, series 4.4, folder 7, CPP.

48. W. W. Keen, "Tribute to S. Weir Mitchell," in *S. Weir Mitchell: Memorial Addresses and Resolutions*, 18; Earnest, *S. Weir Mitchell*, 65–66, 155, 115, 174; "Stotesbury May Be Head of Treasury," *New York Times*, February 22, 1909, 1. S. Weir Mitchell to Mrs. Andrew Carnegie (dated "from my 75th mile stone," perhaps his birthday on February 15, 1904); S. Weir Mitchell to Andrew Carnegie, December 12, 1906; Mitchell to Carnegie, January 16, 1908: all from box 10, series 4.4, folder 4, CPP; Beverly Tucker, *S. Weir Mitchell* (Boston: Richard G. Badger, 1914), 15.

49. Burr, ed., *Weir Mitchell: His Life and Letters*, 392–396. The American Neurological Association (ANA) elected Mitchell to be its founding president in 1874–1875, but Mitchell had to decline the position because of his heavy workload. He became ANA president in 1909 at the age of eighty (Derek Denny-Brown, *Centennial Anniversary Volume of the American Neurological Association* [New York: Springer Publishing Company, 1975], 129–133); James Tyson, "Tribute to S. Weir Mitchell," in *S. Weir Mitchell: Memorial Addresses and Resolutions*, 26–28. Mitchell's largest beneficiary was the College of Physicians of Philadelphia, for which he raised the lion's share of the $365,000 necessary to build a new building in 1906.

50. S. Weir Mitchell to Dr. Simon Flexner, September 4, 1903, box 8, series 4.2, folder 4, CPP; Earnest, *S. Weir Mitchell*, 112; Jacalyn Duffin, *History of Medicine* (Toronto: University of Toronto Press, 1999), 83.

51. Burr, ed., *Weir Mitchell, His Life and Letters*, 220; Carleton B. Chapman, *Order out of Chaos: John Shaw Billings and America's Coming of Age* (Boston: Boston Medical Library in the Francis A. Countway Library of Medicine, 1994); Earnest, *S. Weir Mitchell*, 175.

52. S. Weir Mitchell to Dr. Fielding H. Garrison, September 22, 1913, box 8, series 4.2, folder 5, CPP.

53. Edith Wharton, *Twilight Sleep* (New York: D. Appleton and Co., 1927).

54. S. Weir Mitchell, "Address before the Fiftieth Annual Meeting of the American Medico-Psychological Association, Held in Philadelphia, May 16th, 1894," *American Journal of Psychiatry* 151 (June 1994): 34.

Chapter 2 — The Popular Diagnosis

1. Augustus Hoppin, *A Fashionable Sufferer, or Chapters from Life's Comedy* (Boston: Houghton, Mifflin and Co., 1883), 12, 15–16. Emphasis in the original.

2. F. G. Gosling, *Before Freud: Neurasthenia and the American Medical Community, 1870–1910* (Chicago: University of Illinois Press, 1987), 177–183; G. Alder Blumer, "The Coming of Psychasthenia," *Journal of Nervous and Mental Disease* 33 (1906): 336.

3. Charles Rosenberg has also written on the trope of blaming modern changes for illness, in "Pathologies of Progress: The Idea of Civilization as Risk," *Bulletin of the History of Medicine* 72 (Winter 1998): 714–730. Janet Oppenheim provides

a number of antecedents for neurasthenia in *"Shattered Nerves": Doctors, Patients, and Depression in Victorian England* (New York: Oxford University Press, 1991), 3–109.

4. George Cheyne, *The English Malady; or, A Treatise of Nervous Disease* (London: G. Strahan, 1733), i–ii, 174, 49, 147, 180; Anita Guerrini, *Obesity and Depression in the Enlightenment: The Life and Times of George Cheyne* (Norman: University of Oklahoma Press, 2000), 241–242; Roy Porter, "Nervousness, Eighteenth- and Nineteenth-Century Style: From Luxury to Labour," in *Cultures of Neurasthenia: From Beard to the First World War*, ed. Marijke Gijswijt-Hofstra and Roy Porter (New York: Rodopi, 2001), 31–49; Mark S. Micale, *Hysterical Men: The Hidden History of Male Nervous Illness* (Cambridge, Mass.: Harvard University Press, 2008), 40–43.

5. Thomas Trotter, *View of the Nervous Temperament* (Troy, N.Y.: Wright, Goodenow and Stockwell, 1808; orig. pub. 1807), xii–xiii, iv–v, 13–33. Peter Melville Logan estimated Trotter's book was the first mental health book published in the United States, in *Nerves and Narratives: A Cultural History of Hysteria in Nineteenth-Century British Prose* (Berkeley and Los Angeles: University of California Press, 1997), 16; Micale, *Hysterical Men*, 79–84.

6. Roy Porter explores this concept in "Nervousness, Eighteenth- and Nineteenth-Century Style."

7. G. T. Hayden, *An Essay on the Wear and Tear of Human Life* (Dublin: Fannin and Co., 1846), 45–48.

8. "Brooklyn News," *New York Times*, May 13, 1863, 2; "Died," *New York Daily Times*, May 10, 1854, 8; "Obituary of Hon. David Wilmot," *New York Times*, March 20, 1868, 2; "Bishop Doane's Illness," *New York Daily Times*, October 10, 1852, 4.

9. The Wirz trial was front-page news from the middle of August until his execution on November 11, 1865. See "The Rebel Assassins: Trial of Henry Wirz, the Andersonville Jailor," August 22, 1865, 1; "The Wirz Trial," September 14, 1865, 1; "Postponement of the Trial of Capt. Wirz," September 14, 1865, 1: all from *New York Times*.

10. "The Sudden Illness of Hon. Thomas Ewing," October 24, 1869, 5; "A Fearful Explosion," June 11, 1864, 2; "The Pursuit—The Criticisms on Gen. Meade," July 19, 1863, 4; "State of the City," May 5, 1859, 1: all from *New York Times*.

11. John Whiteclay Chambers II, ed., *The Oxford Companion to American Military History* (New York: Oxford University Press, 1999), 175–176, 742. Numbers on medical personnel serving in the war are imprecise; more than 11,000 doctors served the Union and more than 3,300 served the Confederacy. See George Washington Adams, *Doctors in Blue: The Medical History of the Union Army in the Civil War* (New York: Henry Schuman, 1952), 9; H. H. Cunningham, *Doctors in Gray: The Confederate Medical Service* (Baton Rouge: Louisiana State University Press, 1958), 37. Previous scholars have also made the link between neurasthenia and the professionalization of medicine. See John S. Haller, "Neurasthenia: The Medical Profession and the 'New Woman' of [the] Late Nineteenth Century," *New York State Journal of Medicine* 71 (February 1971): 473–482; Barbara Ehrenreich and Deirdre English, *Complaints and Disorders: The Sexual Politics of Sickness* (New York: The Feminist Press, 1973); Barbara Sicherman, "The Uses of a Diagnosis: Doctors, Patients, and Neurasthenia," *Journal of the History of Medicine and Allied Sciences* 32 (January 1977): 33–54; Gosling, *Before Freud*; Edward Shorter, *A History of Psychiatry: From the Era of the Asylum to the Age of Prozac* (New York: John Wiley and Sons, 1997), 113–144; Andrew Abbott, *The System of Professions: An Essay on the Division of Expert Labor* (Chicago: University of Chicago Press, 1988), 280–314.

12. S. Weir Mitchell, *Wear and Tear, or Hints for the Overworked* (Philadelphia: J. B. Lippincott, 1871). Although the first edition was only 59 pages, later editions of the book reached 76 pages. Future references to *Wear and Tear* will be from the fifth edition (Philadelphia: J. B. Lippincott, 1887; reprint, New York: Arno Press, 1973).

13. Mitchell, *Wear and Tear*, 8, 3, 5, 7; Ernest Earnest, *S. Weir Mitchell: Novelist and Physician* (Philadelphia: University of Pennsylvania Press, 1950), 80; Anna Robeson Burr, *Weir Mitchell: His Life and Letters* (New York: Duffield and Co., 1929), 141.

14. Mitchell, *Wear and Tear*, 5–13.

15. Ibid., 6–10, 34–35, 57–60.

16. Ibid., 12–20, 30–31, 35–58, 62–67. In 1873, Harvard professor of medicine Edward H. Clarke published an influential treatise that argued that girls were not as physiologically suited as boys for competitive education; see *Sex in Education; or, A Fair Chance for the Girls* (Boston: James R. Osgood and Co., 1873).

17. Peter J. Bowler, *Evolution: The History of an Idea* (Berkeley and Los Angeles: University of California Press, 1989), 226–229. As an evolutionary theory, Lamarckism was more popular in America than it was in Europe. In 1889, evolutionary biologist August Weismann helped disprove the Lamarckian theory of inherited acquired characteristics in a gruesome, yet persuasive, experiment in which he cut off the tails of mice for twenty-two successive generations. Lamarckian evolutionary theory of inherited acquired characteristics would suggest that each generation of mice would have slightly shorter tails or no tails at all and Weismann's experiment proved this not to be the case. Nonetheless, Lamarckian evolutionary theories had a home in the American imagination into the twentieth century.

18. M. L. Holbrook, *Hygiene of the Brain and Nerves and the Cure of Nervousness* (New York: M. L. Holbrook, 1878), 52.

19. Mitchell, *Wear and Tear*, 15; Horatio C. Wood, *Brain-Work and Overwork* (Philadelphia: P. Blakiston, Son and Co., 1882); Charles K. Mills, "Mental Over-Work and Premature Disease among Public and Professional Men," in *Smithsonian Miscellaneous Collections*, vol. 34 (Washington: Smithsonian Institution, 1885); Charles K. Mills, "Overwork and Sanitation in the Public Schools of Philadelphia," *Annuals of Hygiene* 1 (1886): 274–278; Mitchell, *Doctor and Patient* (Philadelphia: J. B. Lippincott Company, 1888), 6; H. C. Sawyer, *Nerve Waste* (San Francisco: Bancroft Co., 1888); review of *Nerve Waste* found in "Briefer Notice," *Overland Monthly and Out West Magazine* 12 (July 1888): 111–112; John Harvey Kellogg, *Neurasthenia or Nervous Exhaustion* (Battle Creek, Mich.: Good Health Publishing, 1914); advertisement for *Neurasthenia or Nervous Exhaustion* found in *Lippincott's Monthly Magazine* 95 (April 1915): 133.

20. "Twentieth Century Electrocure," (ca. 1898), box 27; "The German Electric Belts and Appliances," (circa 1888), box 27; "Harness' Electropathic Belt," (circa 1890), box 27; all from the Hartman Center. *Sears, Roebuck Catalogue* (Chicago: Sears, Roebuck and Co., 1902; reprint, New York: Bounty Books, 1969), 476.

21. James Harvey Young, *The Toadstool Millionaires: A Social History of Patent Medicines in America before Federal Regulation* (Princeton, N.J.: Princeton University Press, 1961), 31–43, 93–110. Other important works on the influence of late-nineteenth-century advertising and the development of a modern American culture include Jackson Lears, *Fables of Abundance: A Cultural History of Advertising in America* (New York: Basic Books, 1994), Pamela Walker Laird, *Advertising Progress: American Business and the Rise of Consumer Marketing*

(Baltimore: Johns Hopkins University Press, 1998), and Nancy Tomes, "The Great Medicine Show Revisited," *Bulletin of the History of Medicine* 79 (Winter 2005): 627–663.

22. Young, *The Toadstool Millionaires*, 103; A. C. Cantley, "Some Facts about Making Patent Medicines," *The Chautauquan: A Weekly Newsmagazine* 27 (July 1898): 389; Fred L. Israel, ed., *Sears, Roebuck Catalogue* (Chicago: Sears, Roebuck and Co., 1897; reprint, Philadelphia: Chelsea House Publishers, 1993), 26–32m; Stewart H. Holbrook, *The Golden Age of Quackery* (New York: Macmillan, 1959), 6.

23. William C. Cray, *Miles 1884–1984: A Centennial History* (Englewood Cliffs, N.J.: Prentice Hall, 1984), 19–20; Cantley, "Some Facts about Making Patent Medicines," 389; Young, *The Toadstool Millionaires*, 140–141; "Dr. D. Jayne's Family Medicines and Almanacs for 1876," (Philadelphia: 1875), box 27, Hartman Center.

24. *Dr. Dunlop's Family Practice: A Hand Book of over 100 Common Diseases, Giving Symptoms and Treatment Designed for Family Use* (New York: United States Medicine Co., n.d.), p. 21, box 27, Hartman Center.

25. *Warner's Safe Cure Almanac, 1892* (Buffalo: Cossack and Co., 1891), 36–37; *The Peaceful Life of the Shakers, and The Young Money-Makers of America* (no publishing information available), both from box 27, Hartman Center; Fred L. Israel, ed., *Sears, Roebuck Catalogue*, 1897, 32f.

26. Dr. Miles, "New and Startling Facts for Those Afflicted with Nervous Diseases" (Elkhart, Ind.: Dr. Miles Medical Co., 1891), p. 3, box 29, Hartman Center. Advertising allowed the Miles Medical Company to parlay a demand for neurasthenia medication into a twentieth-century pharmaceutical empire. By 1898, its annual sales had reached $400,000; by 1918 they surpassed $1 million. In 1931, the company developed a new product, Alka-Seltzer, which would supplant Nervine as its best-selling medicine and help drive company sales up to $3.3 million in 1934, a time when the rest of the country was in the grips of the Great Depression. Renamed Miles Laboratories, the company expanded manufacturing to overseas plants, became a Fortune 500 corporation in 1958, and developed such household products as One-A-Day (1940) and Flintstone (1969) vitamins, Bactine antiseptic (1950), and the Morningstar Farms line of cholesterol-free meat substitutes (1973), before merging with the West German pharmaceutical giant Bayer in 1979. That same year, the company reformulated Nervine (which had lingered as an over-the-counter medicine) to remove FDA-prohibited bromide sedatives that, ninety years earlier, were thought to revitalize people's nervous energy. For a history of the company, see Cray, *Miles 1884–1984*.

27. Dr. Miles, "New and Startling Facts"; Dr. Miles, "Treating by Mail: An Illustrative Journal for the People," n.d., pp. 1, 2, box 28, Hartman Center.

28. John Stea and William Fried, "Remedies for a Society's Debilities: Medicines for Neurasthenia in Victorian America," *New York State Journal of Medicine* 93 (February 1993): 120–127; Cray, *Miles 1884–1984*, 3–34.

29. *The Peaceful Life of the Shakers*, 32.

30. *Ibid.*; Dr. Miles, "Honest Words from Honest People," box 27, Hartman Center.

31. For more on the 1922 prohibition of treatment by mail, see Cray, *Miles 1884–1984*, 33; Dr. Miles, "Treating by Mail," 7–8; Sarah Stage, *Female Complaints: Lydia Pinkham and the Business of Women's Medicine* (New York: Norton, 1979).

32. "The Parker Remedy for Men," circular and questionnaire, n.d., box 29, Hartman Center.

33. Dr. Miles, "Honest Words from Honest People."

34. "Suicide of an Alabama Merchant," May 7, 1894, 1; "Leap from the Sixth Story," January 10, 1900, 2; "Lawyer's Leap to Death," January 6, 1901, 3; "Suicide in the Subway," February 19, 1908, 3; "Broker C. W. Whitney Shoots Himself," January 9, 1908, 6: all from *New York Times*.

35. "Suicide of C. J. Vanderbilt," April 3, 1882; "Her Divorce Near, Actress a Suicide," May 8, 1907, 4; "Albert Pulitzer, A Suicide in Vienna," October 5, 1902, 4: all from *New York Times*. For a history of suicide that discusses the stigmatization of the act during the nineteenth century, see George Minois, *History of Suicide: Voluntary Death in Western Culture* (Baltimore: Johns Hopkins University Press, 1999).

36. "Mrs. J. R. Waters Kills Daughter and Herself," May 7, 1906, 1; "Paris Slayer Rich Jersey Landowner," May 30, 1909, C2: both from *New York Times*.

37. "Czarina's Mind Affected," November 30, 1909, 1; "Many Suicides in Russia," February 17, 1909, 1: both from *New York Times*. For a more detailed account of neurasthenia's place in Russian culture, see Laura Goering, "'Russian Nervousness': Neurasthenia and National Identity in Nineteenth-Century Russia," *Medical History* 47 (January 2003): 23–46.

38. "Lloyd Aspinwell Better," June 11, 1893, 13; "Helen Keller Breaks Down," June 25, 1905, 1: both from *New York Times*. "Charles M. Schwab," July 27, 1902, 1; "Charles M. Schwab, Details of Illness," July 28, 1902, 1; "Charles M. Schwab Explains his Condition," July 30, 1902, 6; "Charles M. Schwab Resting in the Mountains," August 19, 1902, 1; "Charles M. Schwab, New York Arrival Interview," August 30, 1902, 1; "Charles M. Schwab Sails for Europe," August 22, 1902, 7; "Charles M. Schwab Working Hard on Voyage," August 29, 1902, 1; "Charles M. Schwab in Italy," October 23, 1902, 9; "Charles M. Schwab at Genoa," November 1, 1902, 9: all from *New York Daily Tribune*.

39. Cyrus Edson, "Do We Live Too Fast?" *North American Review* 154 (March 1892): 281–286.

40. Edson, "Do We Live Too Fast?" 286.

41. Edward Wakefield, "Nervousness: The National Disease of America," *McClure's Magazine* 2 (February 1894): 302–307; "Nerves and Nervousness," *Eclectic Magazine of Foreign Literature, Science, and Art* 122 (February 1894): 278–281; Philip Coombs Knapp, "Are Nervous Diseases Increasing?" *Century Magazine* 52 (May 1896): 146–153; "Domesticated Nervousness," *Scribner's Magazine* 23 (February 1898): 251; "Nervousness and Fatigue in the School Room," *Outlook* 62 (May 6, 1899): 93.

42. William Taylor Marrs, *Confessions of a Neurasthenic* (Philadelphia: F. A. Davis, 1908); Margaret A. Cleaves, *Autobiography of a Neurasthene: As Told by One of Them* (Boston: R. G. Badger, 1910); Charlotte Perkins Stetson, "The Yellow Wall-Paper," *New England Magazine* 11 (January 1892): 647–657; Theodore Dreiser, "Scared Back to Nature," *Harper's Weekly* 47 (May 16, 1903): 816; anonymous, "The Autobiography of a Neurasthenic: The Confessions of a Man Who Had a Nervous Breakdown and Has Tried Many Times to Recover," *American Magazine* 71 (December 1910): 223–231; O. Henry, *Adventures in Neurasthenia: Let Me Feel Your Pulse* (New York: Doubleday, Page and Co., 1910); S. Weir Mitchell, *Roland Blake* (New York: Houghton, Mifflin and Co., 1886); Frank Norris, *The Octopus: A Story of California* (New York: Doubleday, Page and Co., 1901); Edith Wharton, *The House of Mirth* (New York: C. Schribner's Sons, 1905).

43. I. N. Love, "Neurasthenia," *Journal of the American Medical Association* 22 (April 14, 1894): 540; Charles L. Dana, "The Partial Passing of Neurasthenia," *Boston Medical and Surgical Journal* 150 (March 31, 1904): 339–344.

44. Opened in 1883, the dispensary (originally named Morse Dispensary—until 1892, when it was renamed Cooper Dispensary) supported a nervous diseases clinic, headed for over twenty years by Dr. J. O. Hirschfelder.

45. F. Finck, May 3, 1895, vol. 3 (1893–96), 444–445; S. Barver, August 10, 1898, vol. 4 (1896–1900), 363; John Dugan, June 11, 1902, vol. 5 (1900–1904), 311, 516. All from Nervous Disease Cases, CMC.

46. S. Weir Mitchell, "Clinical Lecture on Nervousness in the Male," *Medical News and Library* 35 (December 1877): 177–184; Sidney I. Schwab, "Neurasthenia among Garment Workers," *American Economic Review* 1 (April 1911): 265–270; J. A. Robinson, "Neurasthenia: Its Etiology, Diagnosis, and Treatment," *Journal of the National Medical Association* 4 (January–March 1912): 20–26; Irving Collins Rosse to Frederick Cheever Shattuck, April 22, 1895, FCS-CLM.

Chapter 3 — The Search for Inspiration: Neurasthenia and Therapeutic Spirituality

1. "Bishop Fallows Is a Mind Curist," *New York Times*, December 30, 1907, 1; "How Bishop Fallows Heals the Sick," *New York Times*, January 5, 1908, SM1. Samuel Fallows outlined his views on faith and health in a book he coauthored with his daughter Helen, *Science and Health from the Viewpoint of the Newest Christian Thought* (Chicago: Our Day Co., 1903).

2. Academic studies have identified both destructive and productive effects of neurasthenic introspection. Jackson Lears and Francis Gosling have discussed the harmful, "morbid" introspection that led to depression and emotional paralysis; Gail Thain Parker and Tom Lutz have examined the ways neurasthenic introspection has led to the development of new ways of thinking. See T. J. Jackson Lears, *No Place of Grace: Antimodernism and the Transformation of American Culture, 1880–1920* (Chicago: University of Chicago Press, 1981); F. G. Gosling, *Before Freud: Neurasthenia and the American Medical Community, 1870–1910* (Chicago: University of Illinois Press, 1987); Gail Thain Parker, *Mind Cure in New England: From the Civil War to World War I* (Hanover: University Press of New England, 1973); Tom Lutz, *American Nervousness, 1903: An Anecdotal History* (Ithaca, N.Y.: Cornell University Press, 1991).

3. In arguing that psychotherapy developed out of the late-nineteenth- and early-twentieth-century conflict between physicians and religious healers, this chapter shares much with Eric Caplan's *Mind Games: American Culture and the Birth of Psychotherapy* (Berkeley and Los Angeles: University of California Press, 1998).

4. Julius A. Dresser, *True History of Mental Science* (Boston: Alfred Mudge and Sons, 1887), 10–11; Eva S. Moskowitz, *In Therapy We Trust: America's Obsession with Self-Fulfillment* (Baltimore: Johns Hopkins University Press, 2001), 10–29.

5. Quoted by J. Dresser, *True History of Mental Science*, 8. Emphasis in the original.

6. Beryl Satter, *Each Mind a Kingdom: American Women, Sexual Purity, and the New Thought Movement, 1875–1920* (Berkeley and Los Angeles: University of California Press, 1999), 70–78; Albanese, *A Republic of Mind and Spirit*, 303–313; Larson, *New Thought*, 267–268; Parker, *Mind Cure in New England*, 9; Moskowitz, *In Therapy We Trust*, 10–29.

7. Satter, *Each Mind a Kingdom*, 96, 80; Martin A. Larson, *New Thought; or, A Modern Religious Approach: The Philosophy of Health, Happiness, and Prosperity* (New York: Philosophical Library, 1985), xiii; Catherine L. Albanese, *A Republic of Mind and Spirit: A Cultural History of American Metaphysical Religion* (New Haven, Conn.: Yale University Press, 2007).

8. William James, *The Varieties of Religious Experience* (Cambridge, Mass.: Harvard University Press, 1985), 85; Horatio W. Dresser, *The Power of Silence: An Interpretation of Life in Relation to Health and Happiness* (Boston: G. H. Ellis, 1895), 9.

9. H. Dresser, *The Power of Silence*, 130.

10. Ibid., 14, 47.

11. Larson, *New Thought*, 144–190; Satter, *Each Mind a Kingdom*, 5; Albanese, *A Republic of Mind and Spirit*, 283–329. The exact number of members in the Church of Christ, Scientist, has been debated. Satter used Christian Science's own tallies, which Larson—who is quite critical of Eddy—thought were overinflated; Larson put the number of members in 1906 at no more than fifty thousand.

12. Mary Baker Eddy, *Science and Health, with Key to the Scriptures* (Boston: Trustees under the Will of Mary Baker G. Eddy, 1906), 135, 402. Unless otherwise noted, all future references are to this 1906 edition.

13. Robert Peel, *Mary Baker Eddy: The Years of Trial, 1876–1891* (New York: Holt, Rinehart and Winston, 1971), 161; "Mrs. Stetson's Story of Miss Brush's Will," *New York Times*, February 20, 1901, 1; Eddy, *Science and Health*, 617–618.

14. Albanese, *A Republic of Mind and Spirit*, 299; Satter, *Each Mind a Kingdom*, 66, 271; Regina Markell Morantz-Sanchez, *Sympathy and Science: Women Physicians in American Medicine* (New York: Oxford University Press, 1985).

15. Larson, *New Thought*, 178; Charles Reynolds Brown, *Faith and Health*, 11th edition (New York: Thomas Y. Crowell Co., 1923), 75–125; "Mrs. Stetson's Story of Miss Brush's Will," *New York Times*, February 20, 1901, 1; "Helen C. Brush's Will Ordered Probated," *New York Times*, August 29, 1901, 3.

16. "Death Due to Faith Cure," *New York Times*, June 24, 1899, 2; "Faith Healing Attacked," *New York Times*, April 21, 1900, 9.

17. Charles L. Dana, "Religion and the Nervous Temperament," *New York Times*, February 4, 1900, 23; James Jackson Putnam, "Remarks on the Psychical Treatment of Neurasthenia," *Boston Medical and Surgical Journal* 132 (May 23, 1895): 505, 507–508.

18. Putnam, "Remarks on the Psychical Treatment of Neurasthenia," 505.

19. Sanford Gifford, *The Emmanuel Movement: The Origins of Group Treatment and the Assault against Lay Psychotherapy* (Boston: Boston Medical Library in the Countway Library of Medicine, Harvard Medical School, 1998). Of the 178 patients treated from March through October 1907, 82 suffered from neurasthenia, 24 from generic insanity, 22 from alcoholism, 14 from fears and fixed ideas, 10 from sexual neuroses, 5 from hysteria, and 17 from miscellaneous conditions. See Richard C. Cabot, "New Phases in the Relation of the Church to Health," *Outlook* 88 (February 29, 1908): 504–508. Elwood Worcester to S. Weir Mitchell, January 18 (no year; probably 1909), folder 23, MP-DML.

20. Elwood Worcester, Samuel McComb, and Isador Coriat, *Religion and Medicine: The Moral Control of Nervous Disorders* (New York: Moffat, Yard, and Co., 1908), 4–5; Putnam, "Remarks on the Psychical Treatment of Neurasthenia," 505–511; Eric Caplan, *Mind Games*, 120; Gifford, *The Emmanuel Movement*, 2–3, 60.

21. Worcester, McComb, and Coriat, *Religion and Medicine*, 2, 7–8.

22. Editor, "This Department and the Emmanuel Church Movement," *Good Housekeeping* 44 (March 1907): 405; "Results at Emmanuel," *Good Housekeeping* 45 (November 1907): 504–508; Caplan, *Mind Games*, 123–129; Gifford, *The Emmanuel Movement*, 68.

23. Worcester to Mitchell, January 18 (no year, probably 1909), folder 23, and Worcester to Mitchell, May 5, 1908, folder 26: both MP-DML; "Religion and Ethics: The New Crusade in Behalf of 'Religious Therapeutics,'" *Current Literature* 44 (March 1908): 289–292.

24. Allan McLane Hamilton, "The Religio-Medical Movements," *North American Review* 189 (February 1909): 223–232.

25. S. Weir Mitchell, "The Treatment by Rest, Seclusion, etc., in Relation to Psychotherapy," *The Journal of the American Medical Association* 50 (June 20, 1908): 2036, 2035; Mitchell to Osler, no date, folder 32, MP-DML. Emphasis in the original.

26. Putnam to Worcester, September 12, 1908, box 3, JJPP-CLM; Blow to Putnam, October 10, 1908, box 4, JJPP-CLM.

27. Putnam to Worcester, September 12, 1908, box 3, JJPP-CLM.

28. Ibid.

29. Gifford, *The Emmanuel Movement*, 89–104.

30. Blow to Putnam, June 26, 1910, box 4 (all future references to the Blow-Putnam correspondence are from this box), JJPP-CLM.

31. Biographical information on Susan Blow taken from "Miss Blow Who Put Kindergartens Here, Dies In East," *St. Louis Post-Dispatch*, March 27, 1916, 3; "Miss Susan Blow's Funeral Will Be Held Here Tomorrow," *St. Louis Globe-Democrat*, March 28, 1916, 8; Dorothy Ross, "Susan Elizabeth Blow," in *Notable American Women*, ed. Janet and Edward T. James (Harvard University Press, 1971).

32. Blow to Putnam, March 1, 1894, JJPP-CLM. Although I characterize Blow's relationship with Putnam as friendly, scholar George Prochnik suggested that Blow was deeply in love with Putnam and that the two may have had an affair. See *Putnam Camp: Sigmund Freud, James Jackson Putnam, and the Purpose of American Psychology* (New York: Other Press, 2006).

33. Blow to Putnam, February 12, 1911; March 11, 1910: both in JJPP-CLM.

34. Blow to Putnam, September 17, 1910; December 22, 1903; October 25, 1915; June 15, 1906: both in JJPP-CLM.

35. Blow to Putnam, July 18, 1910; November 24, 1909; July 14, 1907; August 1, 1908; August 19, 1908; November 14, 1909; February 7, 1910; June 26, 1910; April 10, 1914; June 25, 1910; July 30, 1914: all in JJPP-CLM.

36. Putnam to James, June 25, 1910, box 1, JJPP-CLM.

37. Prochnik comes to a similar conclusion in *Putnam Camp*.

38. Jeffrey Sklansky, *The Soul's Economy: Market Society and Selfhood in American Thought, 1820–1920* (Chapel Hill: University of North Carolina Press, 2002), 143–51; Howard M. Feinstein, *Becoming William James* (Ithaca, N.Y.: Cornell University Press, 1984).

39. Blow to Putnam, June 15, 1906, JJPP-CLM.

40. For more on the development of psychotherapy, see Caplan, *Mind Games*, 117–148; Gosling, *Before Freud*.

41. Richard C. Cabot, "The American Type of Psychotherapy," *Psychotherapy* 1, no. 1 (no month, 1908): 5.

Chapter 4 — Neurasthenia, Health, and Gender

1. Oliver Wendell Holmes, *The Autocrat of the Breakfast-Table* (New York: The Heritage Press, 1955, originally published 1858), 40.

2. Michael Kimmel, *Manhood in America: A Cultural History* (New York: Free Press, 1996); Peter Filene, *Him/Her/Self: Sex Roles in Modern America* (Baltimore: Johns Hopkins University Press, 1986); Nancy Cott, *The Bonds of Womanhood: "Woman's Sphere" in New England, 1780–1835* (New Haven, Conn.: Yale University Press, 1977); Mary P. Ryan, *Cradle of the Middle Class: The Family in Oneida County, New York, 1795–1860* (New York: Cambridge University Press, 1981).

3. Catharine Beecher, *A Treatise on Domestic Economy, For the Use of Young Ladies at Home, and At School* (Boston: T. H. Webb, 1842), 34.

4. F. G. Gosling studied the demographics of published neurasthenia cases between 1870 and 1910, and found 154 of the cases involved men patients and 152 involved women patients. F. G. Gosling, *Before Freud: Neurasthenia and the American Medical Community, 1870–1910* (Chicago: University of Illinois Press, 1987), 34.

5. Peter Filene, *Him/Her/Self*; Kimmel, *Manhood in American*; Gail Bederman's *Manliness and Civilization: A Cultural History of Gender and Race in the United States, 1880–1917* (Chicago: University of Chicago Press, 1995).

6. John Reid, September 13, 1893, vol. 3 (1893–1896), 148; Hugh Clyne, November 16, 1892, vol. 2 (1888–1892), 586; Chas Molter, December 22, 1897, vol. 4 (1896–1900), 259; J. O. Moore, June 10, 1896, vol. 4, (1896–1900), 20; S. Barver, August 10, 1898, vol. 4, (1896–1900), 363: all in CMC.

7. Frederic Curran, February 8, 1893, vol. 3 (1893–1896), 22; Jacob Lyne, December 21, 1900, vol. 5 (1900–1904), 110; M. Schlosser, December 3, 1902, vol. 5 (1900–1904), 362: all in CMC.

8. David Corotto, February 8, 1899, vol. 4 (1896–1900), 433; Wm. Oakes, March 29, 1893, vol. 3 (1893–1896), 51: both in CMC.

9. H. Tristram Engelhardt Jr., "The Disease of Masturbation: Values and the Concept of Disease," in *Sickness and Health in America*, ed. Judith Walzer Leavitt and Ronald L. Numbers (Madison: University of Wisconsin Press, 1985), 13–21.

10. Richard Lingeman, *Theodore Dreiser: At the Gates of the City, 1871–1907* (New York: Putnam, 1986); Jerome Loving, *The Last Titan: A Life of Theodore Dreiser* (Berkeley and Los Angeles: University of California, 2005).

11. Theodore Dreiser, *An Amateur Laborer*, ed. Richard W. Dowell, James L. W. West III, Neda M. Westlake (Philadelphia: University of Pennsylvania Press), 4, 12, 17, 39.

12. Theodore Dreiser, *American Diaries, 1902–1926*, ed. Thomas P. Riggio, James L. W. West III, and Neda M. Westlake (Philadelphia: University of Pennsylvania Press, 1983), 81–82, 62, 67–68; Dreiser, *An Amateur Laborer*, 24–25.

13. Dreiser, *American Diaries*, 64, 65.

14. Dreiser, *An Amateur Laborer*, 39, 59.

15. Theodore Dreiser, "Scared Back to Nature," *Harper's Weekly* 47 (May 16, 1903): 816.

16. Dreiser, "Scared Back to Nature," 816.

17. S. Weir Mitchell, *Fat and Blood and How to Make Them* 2nd ed. (Philadelphia: J. B. Lippincott, 1878), 42.

18. Anonymous, "The Autobiography of a Neurasthenic: The Confession of a Man Who Had a Nervous Breakdown and Has Tried Many Times to Recover," *American Magazine* 71 (December 1910): 223–231.

19. "Autobiography of a Neurasthenic," 223–224, 227, 231.

20. Alfred I. du Pont to Frank L. Connable, September 1, 1906, accession 1599, Miscellaneous Papers of Eugene Du Pont (1873–1954), folder 2, The Hagley Museum and Library.

21. Much of the information in this chapter has appeared in David G. Schuster, "Personalizing Illness and Modernity: S. Weir Mitchell, Literary Women, and Neurasthenia, 1870–1914," *Bulletin of the History of Medicine* 79 (Winter 2005): 695–722.

22. *Who Was Who in America* (Chicago: A.N. Marquis Co., 1942), 785; Mount Holyoke College Archives and Special Collections, Mason biographical file (class 1851). Mason also infused episodes from her own life into a biography she wrote for Emily Eames MacVaegh, *Memories of a Friend* (Chicago: Laurence C. Woodworth, 1918).

23. Mason, *Memories of a Friend*, 15.

24. Jane Cunningham Croly, *The History of the Woman's Club Movement in America* (New York: Henry G. Allen and Co., 1898), 60–61; Muriel Beadle, *The Fortnightly of Chicago, The City and Its Women: 1873–1973* (Chicago: Henry Regnery Co., 1973), 3–4; Mason, *Memories of a Friend*, 53, 41–42; Amelia Gere Mason, *The Women of the French Salons* (New York: The Century Co., 1891).

25. Amelia Gere Mason to S. Weir Mitchell, April 25, 1907; Mason to Mitchell, March 17, 1892; Mason to Mitchell, December 6, 1897; Mason to Mitchell, November 10, 1899; Mason to Mitchell, December 28, 1912: all from box 9, folder 7, CPP. All future references to the Mason-Mitchell correspondence come from this box and folder.

26. Mason to Mitchell, 1 April 1900, CPP.

27. Mason, *Memories of a Friend*, 14–15, 57. Maureen Flanagan has also recognized the importance of women in Chicago's reconstruction and the development of a civic culture (Flanagan, *Seeing with Their Hearts: Chicago Women and the Vision of the Good City, 1871–1933* [Princeton: Princeton University Press, 2002]).

28. Mason, *Women of the French Salons*, v–vi.

29. S. Weir Mitchell, *Doctor and Patient* (Philadelphia: J. B. Lippincott, 1888), 139–140.

30. Mason to Mitchell, July 7, 1892, CPP.

31. Regina Markell Morantz-Sanchez, *Sympathy and Science: Women Physicians in American Medicine* (New York: Oxford University Press, 1985).

32. Mason to Mitchell, July 7, 1892, CPP.

33. Mason to Mitchell, March 17, 1892; Mason to Mitchell, December 27, 1886; Mason to Mitchell, July 9, 1912: all in CPP. Emphasis in the original.

34. Ernest Earnest, *S. Weir Mitchell, Novelist and Physician* (Philadelphia: University of Pennsylvania Press, 1950), 73, 130.

35. The best published source on Sarah Butler Wister's life is *That I May Tell You: Journals and Letters of the Owen Wister Family*, ed. Fanny Kemble Wister (Wayne, Penn.: Haverford House, 1979).

36. Kemble Wister, *That I May Tell You*, 3, 7.

37. Mrs. O. J. Wister and Agnes Irwin, eds., *Worthy Women of Our First Century* (Philadelphia: Lippincott, 1877). Although Irwin and Mitchell had opposing views on what constituted the proper education for young women, the two knew each other and kept up a friendly correspondence. Sarah Butler Wister to S. Weir Mitchell, August 18, 1897, series 4.3, box 9, CPP. Subsequent references to the Wister-Mitchell letters come from the same series and box.

38. For an account of Owen Wister Sr.'s career and health, see Steven J. Peitzman, "'I Am Their Physician': Dr. Owen J. Wister of Germantown and His Too Many Patients," *Bulletin of the History of Medicine* 83 (Summer 2009): 245–270. Information on Owen Wister Jr.'s illness can be found in Barbara Will's "The Nervous Origins of the American Western," *American Literature* 70 (June 1998): 293–316. Reference to Wister's sister-in-law comes from Fanny Kemble Wister,

ed., "Sarah Butler Wister's Civil War Diary," *Pennsylvania Magazine of History and Biography* 102 (July 1978): 278.

39. Wister to Mitchell, February 16, 1904 (note that Earnest's biography of Mitchell incorrectly dates this letter as February 6, 1904); Wister to Mitchell, June 19, 1898; Wister to Mitchell, March 23, 1898; Wister to Mitchell, July 29, 1897; Wister to Mitchell, October 13 (no year but most likely 1900, when DaCosta died): all in CPP; Kemble Wister *That I May Tell You*, 11; Carroll Smith-Rosenberg, "The Female World of Love and Ritual: Relations between Women in Nineteenth-Century America," *Signs: Journal of Women in Culture and Society* 1 (Autumn 1975): 5.

40. For a general overview of women's dedication to housework and the physical and mental toll it exacted, see Susan Strasser's *Never Done: A History of American Housework* (New York: Pantheon Books, 1982).

41. Wister to Mitchell, no date (although probably 1896 or 1897); Wister to Mitchell, June 19, 1903: both in CPP.

42. Kemble Wister, "Sarah Butler Wister's Civil War Diary," 290, 296.

43. Historian Daniel Rodgers has found that American workers in the nineteenth century also used neurasthenia as a reason to take breaks from work, while professor of medical anthropology Arthur Kleinman and sinologist Joan Kleinman have found a similar use of neurasthenia, a century later, in late-twentieth-century China. Daniel Rodgers, *The Work Ethic in Industrial America, 1850–1920* (Chicago: University of Chicago Press, 1978), 102–114; Arthur Kleinman and Joan Kleinman, "Somatization: The Interconnections in Chinese Society among Culture, Depressive Experiences, and the Meanings of Pain," in *Culture and Depression: Studies in the Anthropology and Cross-Cultural Psychiatry of Affect and Disorder*, ed. Arthur Kleinman and Byron Good (Berkeley and Los Angeles: University of California Press, 1985), 429–490.

44. Will, "The Nervous Origins of the American Western," 293–316.

45. Wister to Mitchell, September 3, 1893, CPP. Mitchell often prescribed painting to his patients; see *Doctor and Patient*, 167–168.

46. Wister to Mitchell, September 22, 1895, CPP.

47. Virginia Woolf, also a neurasthenic, famously elaborated on this same theme more than thirty years later in *A Room of One's Own* (London: Hogarth Press, 1929) and in *Three Guineas* (London: Hogarth Press, 1938).

48. Wister to Mitchell, August 10, 1897; Wister to Mitchell, September 28, 1903: both in CPP. Carroll Smith-Rosenberg has made similar observations about the role that hysteria played in allowing women to escape, avoid, and redefine their domestic roles. See her essay "The Hysterical Woman: Sex Roles and Role Conflict in Nineteenth-Century America," *Social Research* 39 (1972): 653–678.

49. For works that discuss Gilman's redefinition of women's social roles and household labor, see Beth Sutton-Ramspeck, *Raising the Dust: The Literary Housekeeping of Mary Ward, Sarah Grand, and Charlotte Perkins Gilman* (Athens: Ohio University Press, 2004); Ann J. Lane, *To Herland and Beyond: The Life and Work of Charlotte Perkins Gilman* (New York: Pantheon Books, 1990); Polly Wynn Allen, *Building Domestic Liberty: Charlotte Perkins Gilman's Architectural Feminism* (Amherst: University of Massachusetts Press, 1988).

50. Charlotte Perkins Gilman, *The Living of Charlotte Perkins Gilman: An Autobiography* (New York: Harper and Row, 1963), 8.

51. Ibid., 90–92.

52. Ibid., 92–94.

53. Ibid., 94–95.

54. Ibid., 95–96.

55. Ibid., 96. Part of the folklore surrounding "The Yellow Wallpaper" is that Gilman sent Mitchell a copy of the short story in the hopes that the doctor would read it and make his rest cure more humane. Gilman claims that her strategy worked and that Mitchell modified his therapy on her account. This story, however, is unsubstantiated and sharply questioned by Suzanne Poirier, "The Weir Mitchell Rest Cure: Doctor and Patients," *Women's Studies* 10 (1983): 15–40, and by Julie Bates Dock in *Charlotte Perkins Gilman's "The Yellow Wall-paper" and the History of Its Publication and Reception: A Critical Edition and Documentary Casebook* (University Park: Pennsylvania State University Press, 1998).

56. Charlotte Perkins Gilman, "Through This," *Kate Field's Washington* (September 13, 1893): 166.

57. Charlotte Perkins Gilman, "Making a Change," *Forerunner* 2 (December 1911): 311–315.

58. Charlotte Perkins Gilman, *Women and Economics: A Study of the Economic Relationship between Men and Women as a Factor in Social Evolution* (Boston: Small, Maynard, and Co., 1898).

59. Charlotte Perkins Gilman, "The 'Nervous Breakdown' of Women," *Forerunner* 7 (July–August 1916): 202–206.

60. Maureen Egan, "Evolutionary Theory in the Social Philosophy of Charlotte Perkins Gilman," *Hypatia* 4 (Spring 1989): 102–119; Bederman, *Manliness and Civilization*, 121–169.

61. Grace Peckham, *The Nervousness of Americans: A Paper Read before the American Social Science Association, September 8, 1886* (Boston: Geo. E. Crosby and Co., 1887), 11–12.

62. Jane Addams, "The Subjective Necessity for Social Settlements," reprinted in *Twenty Years at Hull House* (Boston: Bedford/St. Martins, 1999), 89–96, quotations from 92–93. Christopher Lasch talks about Addams, neurasthenia, and women's domesticity in *The New Radicalism in America, 1889–1963: The Intellectual as a Social Type* (New York: W. W. Norton, 1965), 3–68; Gertrude Atherton, "The Woman in Love," *Harper's Bazaar* 44 (May 1910): 305.

63. Mark Adams, *Mr. America: How Muscle Millionaire Bernarr MacFadden Transformed the Nation through Sex, Salad, and the Ultimate Starvation Diet* (New York: Harper, 2009); William Leach, *True Love and Perfect Union: The Feminist Reform of Sex and Society* (New York: Basic Books, 1980); Flanagan, *Seeing with Their Hearts*; Cindy Aron, *Working at Play: A History of Vacations in the United States* (New York: Oxford University Press, 1999); Edward Bellamy, *Looking Backward, 2000–1887* (Boston: Ticknor, 1888).

Chapter 5 — Lifestyle and Managing the Healthy Balance

1. William Taylor Marrs, *Confessions of a Neurasthenic* (Philadelphia: F. A. Davis Co., 1908), 71.

2. According to the *Oxford English Dictionary*, psychologist Alfred Adler originally used the word "lifestyle" in 1929 to describe personality and it was not until the 1960s that the term gained its more recent meaning, associated with choosing how to live one's life.

3. Max Weber, *The Protestant Ethic and the Spirit of Capitalism*, trans. Talcott Parsons (New York: Scribner, 1930).

4. Ellwood P. Cubberley, *Public Education in the United States: A Study and Interpretation of American Educational History* (Boston: Houghton Mifflin, 1934); Lawrence Cremin, *The Transformation of the School: Progressivism in American Education, 1876–1957* (New York: Random House, 1961); Joel Spring, *The American School, 1642–1990: Varieties of Historical Interpretation of the Foundations and Development of American Education* (New York: Longman, 1990).

5. S. Weir Mitchell, *Wear and Tear, or Hints for the Overworked*, 5th ed. (Philadelphia: L. B. Lippincott Co., 1887), 35–47; Dr. Frank Wells, "School Hygiene: Its Relations to the Mass. Emergency and Hygiene Association," *Six Lectures upon School Hygiene, Delivered under the Auspices of the Massachusetts Emergency and Hygiene Association to Teachers in the Public Schools* (Boston: Ginn and Co., 1886), 1–31; Charles K. Mills, "Overwork and Sanitation in the Public Schools of Philadelphia, with remarks on the influence of overwork in the Production of Nervous Diseases and Insanity," *Annals of Hygiene* 1 (September 1886): 275–277. Janet Oppenheim spends a chapter on Critchton-Brown in *"Shattered Nerves": Doctors, Patients, and Depression in Victorian England* (New York: Oxford University Press, 1991), 54–78.

6. H. C. Wood, *Brain-Work and Overwork* (Philadelphia: P. Blakiston, Son and Co., 1882), 70; C. F. Folsom, "The Relation of Our Public Schools to the Disorders of the Nervous System," *Six Lectures upon School Hygiene*, 178–179.

7. "Famous Neurologist Tells Principals and Teachers of Public Schools That They Should Be Diagnosticians," *Philadelphia North American*, February 24, 1904, no page number, series 8.1, box 18, folder 3, CPP; *The Forty-Ninth Annual Report of the Massachusetts Board of Education*, as referred to by Mitchell, *Wear and Tear*, 37–39; Fred W. Atkinson, "The Capacities of Secondary School Students," *School Review* 5 (December 1897): 644.

8. Charles A. Turrell, "Youthful Suicides," *Health* 58 (August 1908): 385–386; Atkinson, "The Capacities of Secondary School Students," 644; Bertha E. Bush, "The Physical Training of Girls," *Christian Advocate* 64 (December 3, 1889): 646.

9. Edward H. Clarke, *Sex in Education; or, A Fair Chance for the Girls* (Boston: J. R. Osgood and Co., 1873); Wells, "School Hygiene," 26; Mitchell, *Wear and Tear*, 43–44, 30–31. Some physicians did not accept Clarke's conclusions that women would suffer mental and physical breakdowns if they competed academically with men. See, for instance, Dr. Grace A. Preston's paper presented before the Massachusetts Medical Society, "Influence of College Life on the Health of Women," *Massachusetts Medical Society, Medical Communications* 16 (January 1, 1893): 165–191. Also, historian Rosalind Rosenberg has written of how Clarke and others who doubted women's academic abilities spurred late-nineteenth-century feminist scholarship in the social sciences. See Rosenberg, *Beyond Separate Spheres: Intellectual Roots of Modern Feminism* (New Haven, Conn.: Yale University Press, 1982).

10. Folsom, "Relation of Our Public Schools to the Disorders of the Nervous System," 168, 181.

11. Dio Lewis, *The New Gymnastics for Men, Women, and Children* (Boston: Ticknor and Fields, 1862; a heavily revised tenth edition was issued in 1868); Mitchell, *Wear and Tear*, 36; Folsom, "Relation of Our Public Schools to the Disorders of the Nervous System," 183.

12. Mills, "Overwork and Sanitation in the Public Schools of Philadelphia," 277; Folsom, "Relation of Our Public Schools to the Disorders of the Nervous System,"

161–193; Dale Allen Gyure, "The Transformation of the Schoolhouse: American Secondary School Architecture and Educational Reform, 1880–1920" (Ph.D. diss, University of Virginia, 2001); Cubberley, *Public Education in the United States*, 604–605; "The Fourth International Congress of School Hygiene," *Science* 38 (August 15, 1913): 224–225.

13. Examples of physicians lecturing teachers include: Frank Wells (addressing Massachusetts teachers, 1884, "School Hygiene"); C. F. Folsom (Physician for Nervous Diseases, Boston City Hospital, addressing Massachusetts teachers, 1884, "Relation of Our Public Schools"); Charles K. Mills (president of the American Neurological Association, addressing the Teachers' Institute of Philadelphia, at the Girls' Normal School, December 11, 1885, "Overwork and Sanitation"); S. Weir Mitchell (addressing public school principals and teachers in Philadelphia, February 24, 1904, "Famous Neurologist Tells Principals and Teachers . . .").

14. Atkinson, "The Capacities of Secondary School Students," 644; Horatio C. Wood, *Brain-Work and Overwork* (Philadelphia: P. Blakiston, Son and Co., 1882).

15. Booker T. Washington, "The Atlanta Exposition Speech" in *Up From Slavery: An Autobiography* (New York: Burt Publishing, 1901), 218–225; Washington, "Afro-American Education," in *A New Negro for a New Century* (Chicago: American Publishing House, 1900), 79–92; Washington, *Working With the Hands* (New York: Doubleday, Page and Co., 1904); R. L. Dabney, "The Negro and the Common School," *The Southern Planter and Farmer* 37 (April 1876): 258.

16. W. E. B. Du Bois, "The Hampton Idea," in *The Education of Black People: Ten Critiques, 1906–1960*, ed. Herbert Aptheker (New York: Monthly Review Press, 1973), 9, 11–12.

17. U.S. Department of the Interior, Bureau of Education, Bulletin, 1916, no. 39, *Negro Education: A Study of the Private and Higher Schools for Colored People in the United States*, prepared in cooperation with the Phelps-Stokes Fund under the direction of Thomas Jesse Jones, specialist in the education of racial groups, U.S. Bureau of Education (Washington: Government Printing Office, 1917), 9, 21–23.

18. John M. Tyler, "How Can We Adapt Our System of Education to Present Needs?" *The School Review* 10 (December 1902): 750–751.

19. C. W. Hackensmith, *History of Physical Education* (New York: Harper and Row, 1966); John Rickards Betts, *America's Sporting Heritage: 1850–1950* (Reading, Mass.: Addison-Wesley, 1974); Peter Filene, *Him/HerSelf: Sex Roles in Modern America* (Baltimore: Johns Hopkins University Press, 1986); Jackson Lears, *No Place of Grace: Antimodernism and the Transformation of American Culture* (New York: Pantheon Books, 1981); Gail Bederman, *Manliness and Civilization: A Cultural History of Gender and Race in the United States, 1880–1917* (Chicago: University of Chicago Press, 1995); Steven A. Riess, *Sports in Industrial America, 1850–1920* (Wheeling, Ill.: Harlan Davidson, 1995); Michael Kimmel, *Manhood in America: A Cultural History* (New York: Free Press, 1996).

20. "College Athleticism," *New York Evangelist* 54 (February 22, 1883): 4; untitled, *Nassau Literary Magazine* 38 (September 1882): 132; "Harvard Foot-Ball War," *New York Times*, November 26, 1883, 2; "Athletic Sports at Harvard," *New York Times*, October 18, 1888, 4; "Football Unfit for College Use: President Eliot Talks of Athletics in His Report on Harvard for Last Year," *New York Times*, January 31, 1895, 6. See also "Dr. Mitchell Scores Present Athletic Craze," *Philadelphia North American*, January 17, 1906, no page available, series 8.1, box 18, folder 3, CPP.

21. Clifford Putney, *Muscular Christianity: Manhood and Sports in Protestant America, 1880–1920* (Cambridge, Mass.: Harvard University Press, 2001), 26–28, 69–71.

22. Wilton Tournier, "Physical Culture for Women," *Godey's Magazine* 127 (October 1893): 462B; Amanda Glesmann, "Reforming the Lady: Charles Dana Gibson and the 'New Girl,'" in *Women on the Verge: The Culture of Neurasthenia in Nineteenth-Century America* (Stanford, Calif.: The Iris and B. Gerald Cantor Center for Visual Arts, 2004), 53–67.

23. "Women Discuss Nervousness," *New York Times*, November 6, 1894, 8; Charlotte Perkins Gilman, *The Living of Charlotte Perkins Gilman: An Autobiography* (New York: Harper Colophon Books, 1975), 94; John S. Haller, "Neurasthenia: The Medical Profession and the 'New Woman' of Late Nineteenth Century," *New York State Journal of Medicine* (February 1971): 473–482.

24. David V. Herlihy, *Bicycle: The History* (New Haven, Conn.: Yale University Press, 2004); Henry Clyde, "Pleasure Cycling," *Current Literature* 17 (June 1895): 10–13; Henry Clyde, *Pleasure-Cycling* (Boston: Little, Brown, and Co., 1895); Martyn [single-word name], "The Universal Bicycle," *New York Observer and Chronicle*, June 25, 1896, 939–940.

25. Clyde, *Pleasure-Cycling*, 18, 148; Keating Wheel Company advertisement, *Current Literature* 17 (June 1895): 13 [capitals in the original]; Dr. Pierce advertisement, *Ohio Farmer* 89 (March 19, 1896): 244; "Now They Are Doctors," *New York Times*, May 9, 1895, 8.

26. Theodore Roosevelt, "The Strenuous Life," in *The Strenuous Life, Essays and Addresses* (New York: Century Co., 1918), 3; Kathleen Dalton, *Theodore Roosevelt: A Strenuous Life* (New York: Alfred A. Knopf, 2002), 89; Theodore Roosevelt to Anna Roosevelt, June 17, 1884, in *The Selected Letters of Theodore Roosevelt*, ed. H. W. Brands (New York: Cooper Square Press, 2001), 35–36; Tom Lutz, *American Nervousness, 1903: An Anecdotal History* (Ithaca, N.Y.: Cornell, 1991), 63–98.

27. "The Strenuous Side of Social Life at Our National Capital," *New York Times*, December 17, 1905, 6.

28. "Root in Training," *New York Times*, August 23, 1907, 1; "Roosevelt Visited Root at Muldoon's," *New York Times*, August 24, 1907, 1; "President Visits Root at Sanitarium," *Los Angeles Times*, August 24, 1907, 14; "Wall Street Talks of Root's Illness," *Los Angeles Times*, August 24, 1907, 14.

29. "The Problem of Finding an Adequate Cure for Our National Malady," *New York Times*, September 1, 1907, SM6; "Root in Training," 1; "Roosevelt Visited Root at Muldoon's," 1; "Gen. Bell Invalid, Army Chief of Staff at Muldoon's," *Los Angeles Times*, October 13, 1907, 11.

30. "Exercise and Rides for Women's Nerves," *New York Times*, September 25, 1910, 14. Charlotte Perkins Gilman used an active health camp for women as the backdrop for her short story "Dr. Clair's Place," *Forerunner* 6 (June 1915): 141–145. Also, see Martha H. Vergrugge, *Able-Bodied Womanhood: Personal Health and Social Change in Nineteenth-Century Boston* (New York: Oxford University Press, 1988); Patricia Anne Vertinsky, *The Eternally Wounded Woman: Women, Doctors, and Exercise in the Late Nineteenth Century* (Urbana: University of Illinois Press, 1994).

31. "Problem of Finding an Adequate Cure for Our National Malady," SM6.

32. Eileen Boris, *Art and Labor: Ruskin, Morris, and the Craftsman Ideal in America* (Philadelphia: Temple University Press, 1986).

33. Reverend John Todd quoted by M. L. Holbrook, *Hygiene of the Brain and Nerves, and the Cure of Nervousness* (New York: M. L. Holbrook, 1878), 240–241; Herbert J. Hall,

"The Systematic Use of Work as a Remedy in Neurasthenia and Allied Conditions," *Boston Medical and Surgical Journal* 152 (January 12, 1905): 29–32; Herbert James Hall to Frederick Cheever Shattuck, January 21, 1905, FCS-CLM; "Handicraft a Nerve Cure," *Los Angeles Times*, November 3, 1908, 114; Susan Hall Anthony, "Dr. Herbert J. Hall: Originator of Honest Work for Occupational Therapy, 1904–1923," (parts 1 and 2), *Occupational Therapy in Health Care: A Journal of Contemporary Practice* 19 (2005): 3–32; Kathlyn L. Reed, "Dr. Hall and the Work Cure," *Occupational Therapy in Health Care: A Journal of Contemporary Practice* 19 (2005): 33–50.

34. Frank Marshall White, "The Occupation and Exercise Cure," *Outlook* 94 (March 12, 1910): 581–582.

35. White, "Occupation and Exercise Cure," 584; Thorstein Veblen, *The Theory of the Leisure Class: An Economic Study in the Evolution of Institutions* (New York: Macmillan, 1899).

36. Cindy Aron, *Working at Play: A History of Vacations in the United States* (New York: Oxford University Press, 1999), 9.

37. "Mt. Clifton, Hedgesville, West Virginia, Season of 1908–09"; "The New Tarrymoore Hotel and Annex, Wrightsville Beach, North Carolina": both from box 47, Hartman Center.

38. The Barker Hotel, *The Gem of the Rockies! Manitou Springs, Colo.; A Brief Description of this Resort, Its Attractions for the Tourist and Advantages for the Invalid* (Manitou Springs: Journal Print, 1885), Beinecke Rare Book and Manuscript Library, Yale (call number Zc49 890ge).

39. Loma Linda Sanitarium, *For Health and Pleasure* (Loma Linda: Loma Linda Sanitarium, 1900), Bancroft Library (call number F869 .L67 .L6). The Loma Linda Sanitarium eventually went bankrupt and was bought for forty thousand dollars by a private party, who then donated it to the fledgling Seventh-day Adventist Church in 1905. That church has since built it into what is today known as the Loma Linda University Medical Center. See Keld J. Reynolds, "Early Days of Loma Linda . . . And Even Before," *Adventist Heritage* 2 (Summer 1975): 42–50.

40. "Miradero Sanitarium, Santa Barbara, California," circa 1901, Bancroft Library (call number pF869 S45 M52).

41. Sheila M. Rothman, *Living in the Shadow of Death: Tuberculosis and the Social Experience of Illness in American History* (New York: Basic Books, 1994), 131–147, 179–225; Emily Abel, *Tuberculosis and the Politics of Exclusion: A History of Public Health and Migration to Los Angeles* (New Brunswick, N.J.: Rutgers University Press, 2007); Southern California Bureau of Information, *Southern California: An Authentic Description of Its Natural Features, Resources, and Prospects* (Los Angeles: Bureau of Information, 1892), 11–12, Bancroft Library (call number F869 S45 M52); G. Wharton James, *Tourists' Guide Book to South California for the Traveler, Invalid, Pleasurist and Home Seeker* (Los Angeles: B. R. Baumgardt and Co., 1894), 440, Bancroft Library (call number F867 J3); Gilman, *Autobiography*, 107.

42. Charles Dudley Warner, *Our Italy* (New York: Harper and Brothers, 1892), 9, 5, 50, 18, 88–89.

43. S. Weir Mitchell, *Nurse and Patient; and Camp Cure* (Philadelphia: J. B. Lippincott, 1877); Mitchell, *Doctor and Patient* (Philadelphia: J. B. Lippincott, 1888), 155–162; Mitchell, *Wear and Tear*, 7–10.

44. "Camping-Out at Rudder Grange," *Scribner's Monthly* 16 (May 1878): 104–105.

45. Barbara Will, "The Nervous Origins of the American Western," *American Literature* 70 (June 1998): 293–316; Owen Wister, "The Evolution of the Cow-Puncher," *Harper's New Monthly Magazine* 91 (September 1895): 606, 608.

46. Robert E. Strahorn, "A Summer Outing on Northwestern Waters," *The Cosmopolitan* 21 (September 1896): 473, 475, 483.

47. Frederick Jackson Turner, "The Significance of the Frontier in American History," in *The Frontier in American History* (New York: Henry Holt and Co., 1920), 37; Turner, "The Problem of the West," in *Frontier in American History*, 211.

48. John Muir, *John of the Mountains: The Unpublished Journals of John Muir*, ed. Linnie Marsh Wolfe (Madison: University of Wisconsin Press, 1979), 234.

49. Stephen Fox, *The American Conservation Movement: John Muir and His Legacy* (Madison: University of Wisconsin Press, 1981).

50. Stanford E. Demars, *The Tourist in Yosemite, 1855–1985* (Salt Lake City: University of Utah Press, 1991), 123; John Muir, "The Wild Parks and Forest Reservations of the West," *The Atlantic* 81 (January 1898): 15–16.

51. John F. Reiger, *American Sportsmen and the Origins of Conservation* (Corvallis: Oregon State University Press, 2001).

52. Fox, *The American Conservation Movement*, 110, 125.

Chapter 6 — The Decline of Neurasthenia

1. Peter Bassoe, "The Origin, Rise and Decline of the Neurasthenia Concept," *Wisconsin Medical Journal* 27 (January 1928): 11.

2. William Broaddus Pritchard, "The American Disease: An Interpretation," *Canadian Journal of Medicine and Surgery* 18 (1905): 10; John E. Donley, "On Neurasthenia as a Disintegration of Personality," *Journal of Abnormal Psychology* 1 (June 1906): 57; Robert T. Morris, *Doctors Versus Folks* (Garden City, N.Y.: Doubleday Page and Co., 1916), 328–329.

3. Jacalyn Duffin, *History of Medicine: A Scandalously Short Introduction* (Toronto: University of Toronto Press, 1999), 58; Douglas VanderHoof, "Diarrhea of Gastric Origin: Diagnosis and Treatment," *American Journal of the Medical Sciences* 144 (August 1912): 172; R. G. Hoskins, "The Interrelation of the Organs of Internal Secretion, part I," *American Journal of the Medical Sciences* 141 (March 1911): 374–385; Hoskins, "The Interrelation of the Organs of Internal Secretion, part II," *American Journal of the Medical Sciences* 141 (April 1911): 535–545.

4. "Activity of Modern Woman a Racial Problem," *New York Times*, August 13, 1911, SM6.

5. Eugene Lyman Fisk, "Prolonging Human Life," *North American Review* 212 (July 1920): 60–61.

6. Rima D. Apple, *Vitamania: Vitamins in American Culture* (New Brunswick, N.J.: Rutgers University Press, 1996); Jacalyn Duffin, *History of Medicine*, 324–327; H. E. Dubin and M. J. Lewi, "The Preparation of a Stable Vitamine Product and its Value in Nutrition," *American Journal of the Medical Sciences* 159 (February 1920): 265; A. L. H., "Vitamines in Corn Silage," *Indiana Farmer's Guide* 31 (March 27, 1919): 27.

7. "Efficiency Test of Domestic Standards for Every Housekeeper," *New York Times*, March 11, 1917, SM4; "Panopepton—Dynamic Food," *American Journal of the Medical Sciences* 157 (March 1919): 5; William C. Cray, *Miles 1884–1984: A Centennial History* (Englewood Cliffs, N.J.: Prentice Hall, 1984); Apple, *Vitamania*, 85–108.

8. James Jackson Putnam, "Remarks on the Psychical Treatment of Neurasthenia," *Boston Medical and Surgical Journal* 132 (May 23, 1895): 505–511; William James, *The Varieties of Religious Experience* (Cambridge, Mass.: Harvard University Press, 1985), 85. Eric Caplan also wrote about this shift in *Mind Games: American Culture and the Birth of Psychotherapy* (Berkeley and Los Angeles: University of California Press, 1998). In a more general sense, this study of the cultural shift toward understanding the human condition through a psychological/psychiatric lens echoes what a number of other scholars have written. See Christopher Lasch, *The Culture of Narcissism: American Life in an Age of Diminishing Expectations* (New York: Warner Books, 1979); Warren Susman, "'Personality' and the Making of Twentieth-Century Culture," *Culture as History: The Transformation of American Society in the Twentieth Century* (New York: Pantheon Books, 1984), 271–285; Edward Shorter, *From Paralysis to Fatigue: A History of Psychosomatic Illness in the Modern Era* (New York: Free Press, 1992); Elizabeth Lunbeck, *The Psychiatric Persuasion: Knowledge, Gender, and Power in Modern America* (Princeton, N.J.: Princeton University Press, 1994); Laura D. Hirshbein, *American Melancholy: Constructions of Depression in the Twentieth Century* (New Brunswick, N.J.: Rutgers University Press, 2009).

9. Frederick Peterson, "Obituary of Dr. Charles Loomis Dana," *Bulletin of the New York Academy of Medicine* 12 (January 1936): 27–30; Charles L. Dana, "Dr. George M. Beard: A Sketch of His Life and Character, With Some Personal Reminiscences," *Archives of Neurology and Psychiatry* 10 (October 1923): 427–435; Charles L. Dana, "The Partial Passing of Neurasthenia," *Boston Medical and Surgical Journal* 150 (March 31, 1904): 339.

10. Dana, "Partial Passing of Neurasthenia," 339–344.

11. G. Alder Blumer, "The Coming of Psychesthenia," *Journal of Nervous and Mental Disease* 33 (1906): 336–338.

12. Blumer, "Coming of Psychesthenia," 336–337.

13. John E. Donley, "On Neurasthenia as a Disintegration of Personality," *Journal of Abnormal Psychology* 1 (June 1906): 55–68.

14. Donley, "On Neurasthenia as a Disintegration of Personality," 56, 66; Blow to Putnam, June 15, 1906, JJPP-CLM.

15. Nathan G. Hale Jr., *Freud and the Americans: The Beginnings of Psychoanalysis in the United States, 1876–1917* (New York: Oxford University Press, 1971), 3–23; Sigmund Freud, *Selected Papers on Hysteria and Other Psychoneuroses*, trans. A. A. Brill (New York: *Journal of Nervous and Mental Disease*, 1909).

16. Sigmund Freud, "On the Right to Separate from Neurasthenia a Definite Symptom-Complex as 'Anxiety Neurosis,'" in *Selected Papers*, 133–154.

17. John E. Donley, "Psychotherapy and Re-education," *Journal of Abnormal Psychology* 6 (April-May 1911): 2; Edward Shorter, *A History of Psychiatry: From the Era of the Asylum to the Age of Prozac* (New York: John Wiley and Sons, 1997), 113–189; Shorter, *From Paralysis to Fatigue: A History of Psychosomatic Illness in the Modern Era* (New York: Free Press, 1992), 233–266.

18. Pearce Bailey, "War Neuroses, Shell Shock, and Nervousness in Soldiers," *Journal of the American Medical Association* 71 (December 28, 1918): 2148–2151.

19. Bailey, "War Neuroses, Shell Shock and Nervousness in Soldiers," 2151–2153; Roy Porter, "Nervousness, Eighteenth- and Nineteenth-Century Style: From Luxury to Labour," *Cultures of Neurasthenia from Beard to the First World War*, ed. Marijke Gijswijt-Hofstra and Roy Porter (New York: Rodopi, 2001), 31–49; Chandak Sengoopta,

"'A Mob of Incoherent Symptoms'? Neurasthenia in British Medical Discourse, 1860–1920," *Cultures of Neurasthenia*, 97–115; Henry Viets, "Shell-Shock: A Digest of the English Literature," *Journal of the American Medical Association* 69 (November 24, 1917): 1779–1786.

20. "Preparing to Care for Shell-Shocked Men," *New York Times Magazine*, June 16, 1918, 62.

21. M. D. Clayton, "When is the Diagnosis of Neurasthenia Justified?" *U. S. Veterans Bureau Medical Bulletin* 1 (January 1925): 61, 64.

22. I. N. Love, "Neurasthenia," *Journal of the American Medical Association* 22 (April 14, 1894): 540; Pritchard, "The American Disease: An Interpretation," 11. For the importance of using a specialized and complex vocabulary to generate professional authority, see Paul Starr, *The Social Transformation of American Medicine: The Rise of a Sovereign Profession and the Making of a Vast Industry* (New York: Basic Books, 1982), 3–29; JoAnne Brown, "Professional Language: Words That Succeed," *Radical History Review* 34 (1986): 33–51.

23. "Secret Nostrums and the Journal," *Journal of the American Medical Association* 34 (June 2, 1900): 1420; "Doctors Assail Patent Medicine Advertising," *New York Times*, October 19, 1905, 6.

24. Samuel Hopkins Adams, *The Great American Fraud: Articles on the Nostrum Evil and Quacks, in Two Series, Reprinted from Collier's Weekly* (United States: P. F. Collier and Son, 1906), 3; "Doctors Assail Patent Medicine Advertising," 6; Starr, *Social Transformation of American Medicine*, 127–134.

25. "The Secret Nostrum vs. the Ethical Proprietary Preparation," *Journal of the American Medical Association* 54 (March 4, 1905): 718–721.

26. "Secret Nostrum vs. the Ethical Proprietary Preparation," 720.

27. "Miles Loses Suit in Equity," *American Druggist and Pharmaceutical Record* 48 (January–June 1906): 177; "Dr. Miles Medical Company vs. the May Drug Company," *Journal of the American Medical Association* 46 (May 12, 1906): 1459–1460.

28. "Miles Loses Suit in Equity," 177; "Dr. Miles Medical Company vs. the May Drug Company," 1459–1460.

29. Starr, *Social Transformation of American Medicine*, 132–133; Herbert W. Hess, "History and Present Status of the 'Truth-in-Advertising' Movement," *Annals of the American Academy of Political and Social Science* 101 (May 1922): 214.

30. Starr, *Social Transformation of American Medicine*, 132;

31. *Dr. Miles Weather Almanac* (1936), 20.

Epilogue: Neurasthenia's Legacy

1. John Schwartz, "Always at Work and Anxious: Employees' Health Is Suffering," *New York Times* (September 5, 2004): 1, 23.

2. There are a number of books about American health, society, and culture that pick up where this one leaves off. See for instance Laura D. Hirshbein, *American Melancholy: Constructions of Depression in the Twentieth Century* (New Brunswick, N.J.: Rutgers University Press, 2009); Elizabeth Lunbeck, *The Psychiatric Persuasion: Knowledge, Gender, and Power in Modern America* (Princeton, N.J.: Princeton University Press, 1994); Eva Moskowitz, *In Therapy We Trust: America's Obsession with Self-Fulfillment* (Baltimore: Johns Hopkins University Press, 2001).

3. George S. Kaufman and Moss Hart, *You Can't Take It With You*, in *Six Plays by Kaufman and Hart* (New York: Random House, 1942), 311–313.

4. Saul Bellow, *Seize the Day* (New York: Viking Press, 1961), 11, 36–37, 42, 47, 45, 73, 88.

5. Albert Abrams, *Nervous Breakdown: Its Concomitant Evils—Its Prevention and Cure—A Correct Technique of Living for Brain Workers* (San Francisco: Hicks-Judd Company, 1901), 3–5; Megan Barke, Rebecca Fribush, and Peter N. Stearns, "Nervous Breakdown in 20th-Century American Culture," *Journal of Social History* 33 (Spring 2000): 565–584.

6. *Dr. Miles Weather Almanac* (1936), 30; F. Scott Fitzgerald, *The Crack-Up*, ed. Edmund Wilson (New York: New Directions, 1945); Diane Disney Miller, "When the Animals Began to Talk," *Saturday Evening Post* 229 (December 8, 1956): 38–39, 79–82, 85.

7. The number of *New York Times* references to *neurasthenia*, *nervous prostration*, *nervous exhaustion*, *nervous breakdown*, *neurosis*, and *psychosis* came from using keyword searches within ProQuest's *Historical New York Times* database. Hits were calculated in ten-year increments.

8. Hans Selye, "A Syndrome Produced by Diverse Nocuous Agents," *Nature* 138 (July 4, 1936): 4; Selye, *The Stress of Life* (New York: McGraw-Hill, 1956), 13, viii, vii.

9. E. H. Van Deusen, "Observations on a Form of Nervous Prostration, (Neurasthenia,) Culminating in Insanity," *American Journal of Insanity* 15 (April 1869): 447; Charlotte Perkins Gilman, "Through This," *Kate Field's Washington* (September 13, 1893): 166; Gilman, "Making a Change," *Forerunner* 2 (December 1911): 311–315; Gilman, "The 'Nervous Breakdown' of Women," *Forerunner* 7 (July–August 1916): 202–206; Abraham Myerson, *The Nervous Housewife* (Boston: Little, Brown and Co., 1920); Betty Friedan, *The Feminine Mystique* (New York: Dell Publishing, 1983), 20–21, 249; Ephraim Rosen, Ronald E. Fox, and Ian Gregory, *Abnormal Psychology*, 2nd ed. (Philadelphia: W. B. Saunders Company, 1972), 161.

10. Donna B. Greenberg, "Neurasthenia in the 1980s: Chronic Mononucleosis, Chronic Fatigue Syndrome, and Anxiety and Depressive Disorders," *Psychosomatics* 31 (Spring 1990): 129–137; Susan E. Abby and Paul E. Garfinkel, "Neurasthenia and Chronic Fatigue Syndrome: The Role of Culture in the Making of a Diagnosis," *American Journal of Psychiatry* 148 (December 1991): 1638–1646; Edward Shorter, "Chronic Fatigue in Historical Perspective," *Ciba Foundation Symposium* 173 (1993): 6–22.

11. Alfred M. Freedman, Introduction to *Before Freud*, by F. G. Gosling (Chicago: University of Illinois Press, 1987), 2; Norma C. Ware and Mitchell G. Weiss, "Neurasthenia and the Social Construction of Psychiatric Knowledge," *Transcultural Psychiatric Research Review* 31 (1994): 101–125; Arthur Kleinman, *Social Origins of Distress and Disease: Depression, Neurasthenia, and Pain in Modern China* (New Haven, Conn.: Yale University Press, 1986).

12. Michael S. Wilkes, Robert A. Bell, and Richard L. Kravitz, "Direct-To-Consumer Prescription Drug Advertising: Trends, Impact, and Implications," *Health Affairs* 19 (March/April 2000): 110–128; Gardiner Harris, "Study Finds Many Doctors Often Give Placebos," *New York Times*, October 24, 2008, 12A; Frank Bass, "AP Analysis Finds that Pain Medication Use Has Risen By 90 Percent," Associated Press State and Local Wire, August 20, 2007; P. Scott Richards and Allen E. Bergin, eds., *Handbook of Psychotherapy and Religious Diversity* (Washington, D.C.: American Psychological Association, 2000).

About the Author

David G. Schuster is an assistant professor of United States history at Indiana University–Purdue University Fort Wayne.

Available titles in the Critical Issues in Health and Medicine series:

Karen Seccombe and Kim A. Hoffman, *Just Don't Get Sick: Access to Health Care in the Aftermath of Welfare Reform*

Leo B. Slater, *War and Disease: Biomedical Research on Malaria in the Twentieth Century*

Matthew Smith, *An Alternative History of Hyperactivity: Food Additives and the Feingold Diet*

Rosemary A. Stevens, Charles E. Rosenberg, and Lawton R. Burns, eds., *History and Health Policy in the United States: Putting the Past Back In*

Barbra Mann Wall, *American Catholic Hospitals: A Century of Changing Markets and Missions*